'It's been a pleasure to read this book and have found it to be an immense resource for work with clients, teaching, in my practice with seniors, and personally. Bernie and Glenys have provided great examples of the benefits of incorporating movement into healthier active lifestyles. Their detailed descriptions of exercises gave me an easy to implement roadmap to get off the couch and get moving!'

Candace Hind, *MSW, RSW, PhD Candidate, School of Social Work, University of Windsor, Social worker/Instructor*

Reintroducing Healthy Movement into Daily Life

This book provides a research-based, user-friendly, practical guide on how to reintroduce movement into our daily lives.

Presenting a rationale for the value of movement to all humans, the book explains why and where movement-based approaches and activities may be used to combat daily stress and promote good mental and physical health. Chapters provide simple, short and easy-to-use ideas and activities, drawing on the authors' combined experience as teachers, coaches, facilitators and therapists. Ideas presented will be applicable to a range of professions and settings such as stay-at-home parents, workers in a factory, shop or office, or professionals in high-stress sedentary jobs.

Reintroducing Movement into Daily Life will be of value to any individual wishing to improve their own health. It also provides guidelines and ideas for professionals working in educational, healthcare and other settings to use with their students/ patients/ clients.

Bernie Warren, PhD, Professor Emeritus, is an internationally respected inter-disciplinary researcher and teacher, and a widely published writer on the arts, education and healthcare, who loves teaching and makes learning *fun!* He has taught in universities worldwide for over 35 years and, since his retirement, has been concentrating on his research and writing.

Glenys McQueen-Fuentes is a movement and physical theatre specialist whose research and interests include movement and music as integral languages across the curriculum and exploring methods for enlivening virtual pedagogy. She has lived and worked for extended periods in France, New Zealand and Mexico.

Reintroducing Healthy Movement into Daily Life

Combating Stress, Disease and Ill Health

Bernie Warren and Glenys McQueen-Fuentes

Routledge
Taylor & Francis Group
LONDON AND NEW YORK

Designed cover image: © Getty Images

First published 2023
by Routledge
4 Park Square, Milton Park, Abingdon, Oxon OX14 4RN

and by Routledge
605 Third Avenue, New York, NY 10158

Routledge is an imprint of the Taylor & Francis Group, an informa business

British Library Cataloguing-in-Publication Data
A catalogue record for this book is available from the British Library

Library of Congress Cataloging-in-Publication Data
A catalog record has been requested for this book

ISBN: 978-1-138-34228-6 (hbk)
ISBN: 978-1-138-34230-9 (pbk)
ISBN: 978-0-429-43980-3 (ebk)

DOI: 10.4324/9780429439803

Typeset in Times New Roman
by Taylor & Francis Books

Contents

Figure

Contributors

Professor Emeritus Bernie Warren, PhD, studied dance-movement and drama-theatre in the UK, Europe, Canada and the United States; worked as an actor, dancer, choreographer and director; and was the founder of Fools For Health – working in hospitals and healthcare facilities as Dr Haven't-a-Clue.

Prior to coming to Canada in 1982 he taught drama and dance in schools throughout the UK and Ireland. For more than 35 years he held positions within both drama/theatre and psychology, and taught courses – in acting, devised theatre, drama therapy, educational drama, movement and voice – at universities and colleges around the world.

He is an internationally respected researcher and teacher on the role of the arts in healthcare and education and the author of numerous books. In 2001 he was awarded the University of Windsor's Alumni Award for Distinguished Contributions to University Teaching and in 2009 the University of Windsor's Outstanding Faculty Research Award (Established Scholars/ Researchers). He has been included in *Canadian Who's Who* since 1994.

He recently retired from full-time teaching at the University of Windsor as Professor Emeritus. Since his retirement he has been concentrating on his research and writing; and on teaching short courses for professional organisations and at various universities around the world. His most recent book, *Teddy Teaches Tai Chi* (an illustrated book for children), will be published by YGTMama Media in August 2022.

Glenys McQueen-Fuentes is a movement specialist with degrees from McGill University (BA Drama), Jacques Lecoq's École Internationale de Théâtre du Mouvement in Paris, France, and Brock University (MEd). She spent a year in New Zealand as a founding member of the group Theatre Action, performing and teaching in colleges, on teacher training programmes and for theatre companies. Theatre Action represented New Zealand at the South Pacific Trade and Cultural Fair in Suva, Fiji.

She then spent 11 years teaching movement, performing and coaching (non-verbal theatre styles) in professional theatre in Mexico City with UNAM's University Theatre Centre (CUT), Teatro Epico and Las Sombras Blancas, who did extensive applied theatre work in poor areas throughout Mexico City. She also worked with CONASUPO's Teatro Campesino.

In Canada, as Associate Professor, Department of Dramatic Arts at Brock University, she taught and directed for thirty years. Her areas of expertise included physical and international theatre forms, drama in education and applied theatre. While at Brock she presented hundreds of workshops for teachers (grades 1–12).

She recently retired from full-time teaching but continues as Co-director of DramaSound Projects, exploring effective use of movement, drama and music for teaching, learning, creativity, leadership and community building in all areas of education, health and business.

Acknowledgements

We want to thank everyone at Routledge/Taylor & Francis who have worked with us on this project; but most particularly Joanne Forshaw, who started the ball rolling, and Grace McDonnell for helping us finish it.

I (GMF) would like to thank friends, students, colleagues and places for support and inspiration! For modeling creativity as a given for all, thanks to my parents, Georgina Boux, Melissa Elsie, Fariya Doctor, Christine Boyko-Head, Katya Davison, Robin Patterson – and of course, Jacques Lecoq. And a hats-off thanks to Bernie Warren, whose patience, humour and role-modeling continue to inspire!

And to Gato, for continuous creative-critical intuition and advice that is always, always right!

I (BW) would like to thank all the dancers at LUDUS Dance in Education during my time there (1980–82), especially Chris Thompson and Lesley Hutchison; and my students, colleagues and teachers, especially Yon, Master Hu and George Mager. I learned so much from all of you.

I also would like to thank Glenys McQueen Fuentes for making the extremely long journey to complete this book memorable and enjoyable.

Most importantly I want to thank Dr Fraud for her support and perceptive insights, and for not closing the door to my office loudly when I was on the phone passionately discussing the book.

An Introduction To The Book And Its Authors

Always Moving

Our Lives Are Enmeshed In Story

We are all the heroes of our own tales. We exist through the way that we talk about ourselves, and the way others talk about us when we are not there. Our life's narrative unfolds moment by moment through the actions and decisions that we make in every situation. We are described and discussed through these actions as perceived and analysed by others.

How we speak about ourselves affects our sense of self and affects how others think of us. We cannot control others' responses to our behaviour, but we can control our own responses to other's actions and views of us. Stories about us continue when we are not there and may linger long after we die.

The story of the authors of this book begins with the fact that we are always moving. Over the course of our careers (at the time of writing we have 90+ years' professional practice between us), we have taught physical theatre and dance in schools and universities and employed movement experiences across the lifespan in hospitals and healthcare facilities, with community groups and business professionals. Throughout our careers people constantly commented on our energetic approach to life; that we always seemed to have multiple projects on the go. Yet while we share many traits and attributes, we are very different people – in both our training(s) and our experiences.

The Road To Here: Bernie

I (BW) was born with, or acquired, ADD/ADHD. I was *always* moving. I was placed on Ritalin at 18 months old – although the family story is that my dad (a pharmacist) medicated me so I didn't interrupt my parents having sex!

As I grew up, I became a moving actor/dancer and martial artist and for the past fifty years I have studied many different styles of movement with a wide range of teachers. Along the way I taught classes and workshops for:

- Professional dance and theatre companies in the UK, Canada, and around the world.

DOI: 10.4324/9780429439803-1

- Children and adults of all ages and abilities, not only in classrooms but also in non-traditional settings worldwide.
- Children and adults with life-changing and life-threatening conditions.

Now

My daily martial arts practice, in particular Qigong,[1] and more recently some Yoga,[2] has in large part:

- Removed all symptoms of my hyperactivity disorder.
- Made my ADD in large part manageable *without* medication.
- Helped me overcome my fear of water – I have finally learned to swim.

At some point, influenced in large part by my late friend Yon,[3] I have realized that *all* my teachings are based on:

- Eastern philosophies, particularly Taoist and Buddhist teachings.
- Breathing techniques – *how we breathe* is the basis for, and affects, how we move and everything we do.

My approach in the last few years, as any of my students will tell you, has been simplified to:

Breathe. Smile. Move.

My journey in movement has taught me:

- How to simply adapt exercises and ideas to the ability level of each participant.
- How to use language to enable individuals to successfully participate in the activities.
- To see the connections between things and that all things are connected

The Road To Here: Glenys

Unlike Bernie, I had no ADD or ADHD. However, I was always active in the extreme, and sat down or stopped only under duress.

Major Formative Movement Influences

Between age ten and 18, my local YMCA provided me with a lifelong model for teaching, leadership, and creativity. As 'Y' leaders, we were 'taught to teach' gymnastics, games, dance, fitness, and aquatics to infants through to adults, with and without disabilities. We attended (and often organized) conferences, competitions, and leadership camps. We were expected to be responsible and enterprising – so we were.

My parallel interests in theatre, movement, sports, and dance continued throughout high school – again, with camps, competitions, and ongoing workshops. At university, after learning of a theatre style combining movement and multiple non-verbal performance forms, I followed graduation with two years of post-graduate studies at the Jacques Lecoq International School of Physical Theatre in Paris, France.

After Lecoq, with four classmates I spent a year in New Zealand as a founding member of Theatre Action – creating shows, performing, teaching, and touring.

From there, I spent 11 years teaching, coaching, and performing (movement and non-verbal theatre techniques) in Mexico City with the National Autonomous University of Mexico (UNAM)'s professional school and performance centre, the CUT, as well as with and for numerous other groups.

In Canada, with Rafael Fuentes, my composer husband, I co-founded DramaSound Projects, and focused my teaching, directing, and research on increasing the use of movement and music in the arts, theatre, education, and daily lives.

Transition To Now

- Despite an overall positive environment, the creative, most demanding area of my pre-retirement workplace required continuously interacting in a toxic, destructive situation that I could not escape or alter.
- I handled the situation badly and ended up forty pounds heavier and with an array of health problems.
- My mobility became so compromised that I was assigned a TA to demonstrate in my movement classes.
- Then I ran into an 'I hate movement' friend, who had been working with a personal trainer to alleviate health issues. She had transformed into an energetic, slimmed-down, *healthy* version of herself.
- I met her trainer and began my own journey – which I call my 'Body/Movement PhD' – back to lowering or eliminating my abovementioned physical problems.
- I was shocked by how far research had come in altering many basic 'good movement' daily practices, and the extent to which some of my own habits were contributing to my mobility and health problems rather than solving them.
- NB: while my 'fitness' program has a Western 'edge', my trainer, Melissa Elsie, is holistic in her approach, constantly expanding her research and knowledge base and developing her own extremely creative approaches.
- My *now* involves holistic fitness exploration, including 'full-body breathing', "rolling", and fascia-releasing techniques, all of which keep me mobile, agile, and pain free.

- I also attend classes with Fariya Doctor, a talented Feldenkrais practitioner in my area. I am always astounded by the brilliance of Feldenkrais' work on (re)connecting the brain and the body in surprisingly simple, often instantly effective ways. The neuroplasticity of the brain – its ability to find 'new avenues' for the body to mobilise – is the basic experience of each class. Exhilarating, freeing, and hope-giving for future advances.

On Not Meeting And Working Together

Glenys apparently heard about me in 1983 when she was working at University of Alberta, while I (BW) first heard about Glenys in 1986 when I was teaching at Concordia University in Montreal. Michael Thomas, the Drama and Arts Advisor for the English School board, told me that I really should meet her as we would have a lot in common. However, we didn't meet for another twenty years. We kept just missing one another but admiring each other's work from afar!

We finally met and started to work together in 2007. After this first meeting we visited each other's university to teach movement classes as guest lecturers. About 12 years ago we started to discuss writing a book together. Originally the book was going to simply be a handbook, a guide to teaching movement in schools, colleges, and universities and to performing artists. This book is still waiting in the wings. However, as we were considering what to write together, we started to discuss our work in movement for health.

Why Did We Decide To Write This Book?

Over several years we read many different articles about the rising epidemic of mental and physical ill health and disease, which we believe is caused in large part by inactivity and poor lifestyle choices. These articles made us greatly concerned about people being far too sedentary while dealing with financial, family, and job-related stresses, leading to increased use of drugs and alcohol and a rise in obesity, heart disease, type-2 diabetes – a reduction in physical education programs only compounding these problems

These problems have been exacerbated over the last few years by the Covid-19 global pandemic. The sedentary stresses of online learning and zoom meetings set up by educators/business leaders, etc., in response to Covid protocols did not include movement breaks or any encouragement for adjusting body/work habits to that reality.

We realised that we had a wealth of practical information, ideas, and exercises related to these topics. Our discussions led us to the conclusion that we needed to share our knowledge and the skills we have acquired, through what colleagues describe as our distinguished careers, regarding the value of movement and its role in our health. We decided to write this book in the hope it would help individuals take more control over their lives

We discussed our movement experiences and the various styles we have experienced in our many years working in dance-movement education and training. We talked about our own preferences for some styles, and, irrespective of our personal feelings, the different benefits each of these movement forms has for the participant.

As we continued to write, constantly comparing notes, we became aware that there are certain similarities and points of connection as well as points of difference in our practice and experiences.

It also became clear that it was not always possible to merge our two styles, and so we allowed them to stand side by side. We started from the premise that Glenys' baseline movement worldview is Lecoq-based, while mine (BW) is rooted in Laban analysis and traditional Eastern breathing practices found in Yoga and Qigong. Glenys is influenced by Lecoq's emphasis on *action, movement images, metaphors and poetics*, while I am influenced by Laban's emphasis on *movement analysis* and the Eastern focus on *natural images and metaphors*. We also accepted that these 'baselines' affect how we each describe movement.

However, as we journeyed further together, we discovered that the references to and use of natural images and metaphor, so prevalent in the Eastern focus that is Bernie's background, are also cornerstones of Lecoq's approaches to movement analysis, exploration, and performance creation that Glenys emphasises. We both speak often of nature and of natural occurrences and processes in our writing. And we both use Laban for movement analysis – albeit differently, both quantitatively and qualitatively. Bernie puts the emphasis on Laban's approach to movement analysis through descriptive words (qualities, shapes, efforts, etc.). He understands it profoundly and can use Laban as a 'trampoline' or 'springboard'. Glenys uses Laban's words for analysis – but only as a post-action reflection for deepening image observational work to enhance actions and analysis.

At the end of the day, we are different. We have had different life experiences, think differently, and write differently but we do have a shared vision. So, throughout this book we have tried to find a common ground, to speak as much as possible with one voice in an attempt not to confuse you, the reader.

The Heart Of The Matter: What This Book Is About

The central theme of this book is that reintroducing movement into one's daily life helps combat stress, disease, and conditions of ill health and promotes good physical and mental health, improved quality of life, and a sense of wellbeing.

Reintroducing Healthy Movement provides explanations of research and evidence-based best practice, written in a user-friendly style that seeks to enable readers to make positive changes in their daily lives and/or their professional practice.

It provides a rationale for the value of movement to all humans. It explains why and where movement-based approaches and activities may be used to combat daily stress and promote good mental and physical health and provides simple, short, and easy to use ideas and activities that may be carried out at work, even while standing or at a desk.

This book will be of value to *any* individual wishing to improve their own health – whether a stay-at-home parent, a worker in a factory, shop, or office, or a professional in a high-stress sedentary job. It is our strong belief that adding healthy movement into our lives helps us change our narrative. To perhaps write a story that we prefer, one that is longer, happier, and healthier.

Notes

1 Qigong describes a group of physical, mental, and spiritual practices that originated in Ancient China. It focuses on cultivation of internal energy through physical exercises which center on breathing patterns, physical posture, and coordination to stimulate hormone secretion, promote immune function and oxygenation of body cells.

2 Yoga describes a group of physical, mental, and spiritual practices that originated in Ancient India.

Yoga *āsanas* incorporate stretching and breathing and can help improve a person's physical and mental wellbeing. Regular Yoga practice of *āsana* and meditation helps create mental clarity and calmness; increases body awareness; relieves chronic stress patterns; relaxes the mind; centres attention; and sharpens concentration.

NB Yoga is an ancient spiritual discipline and in our opinion demands the respect of capitalisation, hence the styling throughout.

3 Yon worked for over twenty years at Dartington College of Arts, Totnes, Devon, where he taught acting-directing and voice music. His work bridged the boundaries between dance, drama, and music and he employed his innovative and eclectic style of working with a broad spectrum of people, covering a wide range of ages and abilities.

Part I

The Value Of Movement

In the four short chapters within this section the authors explore the value of movement to health and personal development and to staying healthy throughout one's lifetime.

DOI: 10.4324/9780429439803-2

Chapter 1

The Value Of Movement To Healthy Development

Play Is The Thing

All mammals play, and more than this they need to play to learn. Play itself is unique and individual but short-lived. Whereas a game (often considered a universal teaching medium) has rules that are transportable and is sufficiently systematic that it may be repeated by others in other places.[1]

The effects and knowledge gained from play may be essential to healthy development and long lasting. Some authors suggest that play is the principal instrument of growth and that without play there would be no *normal* adult cognitive life.

All Play Involves Creativity, Imagination, Movement … And Fun

For all of us, our body is our instrument of expression and exploration. It is one of the primary ways through which we tell and inhabit the developing story of our lives.

In childhood it is through the movement of our bodies that we start to build a picture of our world. As we develop, we explore our capabilities and start to learn what our bodies can do.

This exploration and movement of our body parts leads to a growing awareness of our body's structure and to the growth of our body image. Not only is this early physical exploration important to the developing self-concept of young children but also throughout life this testing and usage of our bodies is linked to cognitive, physical, and psycho-social development, particularly in the areas of health and wellbeing.

This development comes with a few caveats:

- *New tasks/activities can be very threatening* as they require the acquisition of new social rituals.
- *Fear of the unknown* is a major factor in the learning of new performance skills.
- *People, especially children, need security*, and on some occasions the new skills being learned are so terrifying that we withdraw or return to old behaviours.

DOI: 10.4324/9780429439803-3

- *Children may indulge in antagonistic behaviour* prior to indulging in new activities, which are not only to their benefit but which they may ultimately enjoy.
    a Some children require ritualistic behaviour prior to their involvement in learning new tasks.
- *Skill is attained and retained only with practice* – without the opportunity to practise, skills are difficult to master, and they atrophy without regular use.

Skill Areas Developed Through Movement Play and Games[2]

The way one plays has been seen by psychologists as a measure of psychological integration and has given rise to the development of play therapy.[3]

There are many psychological interpretations of reasons for play. We would suggest that there are four major areas where play in all its forms is of 'functional value' to human beings:

- *Playing with objects* – babies start by touching and tasting objects
- *Skill acquisition* – e.g., tag games, leapfrog
- *Socialisation* – especially through imitation/rehearsal e.g., hunting games, teacher/pupil/school games
- *Cognitive development* – playing with ideas.

In general, it is through play that we learn to

- Explore the world, and
- Learn about ourselves in relation to others.

Angela Henderson has written a great blog which explores this in more depth, suggesting there are four major benefits of play for children.

Social integration:

- Acquiring skills necessary to good social functioning;
- Building cooperation and trust with peers; and
- Understanding the rules of social performance or generally improving social interactions:
    a Social competence
    b Temperament
    c Sense of humour.

Creativity and self-expression:

- Developing expressive and receptive language;

- Encouraging sensory awareness; and
- Enhancing imagination, spontaneity, and abstract thought.

Body awareness and physical control:

- Acquiring physical dexterity and control;
- Developing awareness of body schema and body image;
- Providing outlets for emotional and physical energies; and
- Practising impulse control.

Cognitive skill development:

- Enhancing memory and recall;
- Developing concentration;
- Encouraging reflectivity;
- Practising anticipation of consequences; and
- Comprehending and solving problems.

Embodied Knowledge

> Bodies hold history, memory, thought, feelings, and desires. Bodies hold language and silence. Our bodies are repositories of knowledge, but these knowledges are not always knowable in and through language – they can be felt, imagined, or dreamed.[4]

Embodied knowledge describes something we know 'in our bones' without having to think about it. Moreover, we may not even know how we know it, we just do. It is why we can accomplish repetitive movements without thinking about them.

Embodied learning helps individuals do without thinking, analysing, reflecting, discussing –we just perform the necessary action to negotiate our world. This is especially important if when driving we encounter a road incident that requires a spontaneous reaction to avoid crashing or hitting a pedestrian.

> Do not ask how intelligent I am but rather how I am intelligent.[5]

When I (BW) was much younger I used to argue a *lot* with my father, a brilliant if somewhat underachieving man, who read voraciously on almost every subject! At the time it seemed to me he used to challenge almost every statement I made with "where did you get *that* from?" Now, as I look back, I realise all that back and forth arguing has made me as an academic try whenever possible to document and footnote where I *did* get 'that' from.

As an adolescent it was extremely stressful to me, but as I have become older, and I hope wiser, I realise that much of what I knew was embodied learning – ideas and other 'facts' I discovered not just from reading books and articles and scientific papers, but through tactile-kinaesthetic knowledge gained from openly interacting with the world.

Embodied knowledge is essential to movement experiences and all creative activities. It touches on a concept I (BW) have explored in several other works, the heart of the creative process being the relationship between liminal states[6] and creative moments.[7]

Embodied Learning And Neuroplasticity

This process of *embodied learning* is tied at least in part to *neuroplasticity*[8] in the brain. Until recently, scientists believed that the brain stopped growing around the age of 16. But current research suggests that the brain can continue growing and changing throughout the lifespan, refining its structure or shifting functions to different regions of the brain.

The importance of neuroplasticity can't be overstated: It means that it is possible to change dysfunctional patterns of thinking and behaving and to develop new mindsets, new memories, new skills, and new abilities. It is suggested that movement activity and embodied learning are intrinsically linked to neuroplasticity.

Notes

1 In his seminal book Man Play and Games (1961), Roger Callois suggested that:

- *Play* is free, separate, uncertain, and unproductive, yet regulated and make-believe.
- A *game* is a specialised form of play: one that has order and structure – a beginning, middle, and end.

More simply put, games have rules that must be followed, while play has rules that are malleable and/or changeable and unlike a game has no predetermined end.

2 A. Henderson (2022), www.finleeandme.com.au/understanding-the-benefits-of-play-for-our-children/

3 V. Axline (1947), *Play Therapy* (New York: Ballantine Books).
See also: www.counseling.org/resources/library/ACA%20Digests/ACAPCD-12.pdf

4 P. Stein (2004), 'Representation, Rights, and Resources: Multimodal pedagogies in the Language and Literacy Classroom', in *Critical Pedagogies and Language Learning*, ed. B. Norton and K. Toohey (New York: Cambridge University Press).

5 In his book *Frames of Mind* (1983), Howard Gardner first put forward his theory of multiple intelligence, which he sorted into seven types: logical-mathematical; spatial; tactile-kinesthetic; musical; verbal; Interpersonal; and introspective. These later became known as 'the seven dwarfs'.

6 Liminal state: A term adapted from social anthropology. It was originally applied to rites of passage. Limen means a threshold and a liminal act applies to a rite of passage where the participant passes over an actual or metaphorical threshold.

Liminal state is sometimes referred to in the West as "flow" or in the East as "no mind". It is an 'altered' state, which describes the moment when intellectual, emotional, physical, and spiritual aspects of one's being are in harmony.

7 Creative moment: A liminal state that brings together physical, intellectual, emotional, and spiritual aspects of our being in a way that offers unique opportunities for transformation to take place.

8 Neuroplasticity is the brain's capacity to continue growing and evolving in response to life experiences. This capability suggests a glimmer of real hope to everyone from stroke victims to dyslexics. For more information, see www.psychologytoday.com/us/basics/neuroplasticity.

Chapter 2

Movement Is Everywhere And In Everything We Do

All Things Dance

> Dance is a series of frozen images
> moved through time and space by emotion and /or rhythm.

There is movement in everything we do. As you sit or stand reading this book, you are breathing, your eyes are scanning the page, so even though you are sitting or standing still, your body is moving. As you tie your shoelaces or drink your coffee you are constantly moving.

Everywhere we go there is movement! Be it cars on a road or the wind rustling the trees – where there is life there is movement. For *all* living organisms – and, one can argue, many inanimate objects – are constantly involved in a dance of sorts with their environment. Movement is integral to our lives as we grow physically and emotionally as human beings. Creative movement that is purposeful is perhaps even more important.

The body is the way we express ourselves, communicate, and make connections with others. Body movement can increase self-worth and deepen a sense of self-awareness, thus allowing an individual to gain a greater appreciation of human interaction. By exploring the life of objects and of other people we expand our own movement vocabulary. Through this process we gain insight into our self and our environment.

By embodying another being we can create a mode of knowledge unattainable through mere words. By literally imagining putting oneself in another's shoes – moving as this other person, animal, or object – we can learn more about how they feel and why they move and act that way, encouraging empathy. Moreover, it provides an individual with a mirror to their true self – an insight into who we are as human beings.

Movement is a way in which we may learn and make sense of information that can't be processed through words and thoughts alone. Our body holds information that our brain is either not aware of or can't make sense of. One example is so-called "muscle memory"[1]; another is the work of Dr Ida Rolf and her system of Rolfing, which focuses on releasing,

DOI: 10.4324/9780429439803-4

realigning, and balancing the whole body to help restore flexibility and revitalize energy.[2]

Movement is a key component in finding this information, ridding our body of trauma, and building a connecting path for information to our brain. Creative movement that is purposeful is perhaps even more important as it provides an opportunity for each of us to take a little control of how our life unfolds.

Only One Body – Many Ways Of Moving

Same, But Different!

No two bodies are the same! However, while there are obvious exceptions (e.g., genetic malformations, structural abnormalities, and reduced ability caused by various forms of traumatic injury), we all have basically the same architecture and structure. For notwithstanding these 'outliers', most human beings have basically the same anatomy.

Anyone who dances, runs, walks, or practices martial arts –or, frankly, does any land-based movement – is aware of their knees, hips, and ankles and how at some point in their life they are likely to 'injure' these joints in some way. This risk of injuring them increases with weight gain and age.[3]

The Influence Of Laban And Lecoq On Western Movement

As mentioned earlier, we have each studied the work of Jacques Lecoq and Rudolf Laban, the two major influences on the teaching of dramatic movement – with Glenys' work being primarily based on the work of Lecoq and Bernie's on Laban.

Rudolf Laban uncovered the basic principles of movement structure and purpose. He created *Labanotation*, a clear and concise language for describing human movement applying his theories to many areas – from the performing and visual arts to education to efficiency studies of factory workers. His influence on dance performance and choreography, theatre, dance/movement therapy, and visual art was substantial.

Jacques Lecoq was a French stage actor and acting movement coach. He was best known for his teaching methods in physical theatre, movement, and mime, which he taught at the school he founded in Paris known as École internationale de Théâtre Jacques Lecoq. His influence on the world of mime, physical theatre, and clowning is immense.

There are many points of congruence between the approaches of these influential teachers, but as Glenys likes to say, the differences may be summed up by, "Laban's work centres on words, while Lecoq's centres on image(s)."

Movement Analysis[4]

There are several ways one can analyse movement. Here we present a couple of ways that we have each used extensively.

Range Of Movement

The body is capable of a wide range of movement, but all movement can be broken down into five basic actions. This kind of breakdown is known as a movement analysis. The five basic actions are:

- *Travel*: redistribution of weight through space
- *Balance*: stillness in equilibrium
- *Turn*: rotation around an axis
- *Jump*: launching weight into the air
- *Gesture*: movement without change of weight usually of a limb or limbs around the torso.

Further, in this simple form of analysis, the body is capable of three kinds of mechanical action:

- Bending,
- Stretching
- Twisting.

Quality Of Movement

Laban considered that the quality of any movement can be described by four movement factors:

• SPACE	high–low	near–far
• WEIGHT	light–strong	soft–hard
• TIME	fast–slow	sudden–sustained
• FLOW	free	bound

As well as these elements, all movements involve one or more parts of the body, have a direction, and are executed in relation to other people or objects. In addition to the words that describe movement actions and qualities, there are some basic descriptors, which may be useful in planning, running, or describing any movement activity. Simple language to describe and analyse movement can be found in the *How We Move* table at the end of the chapter.[5] We have also included an alternate way of analysing movement.[6]

These ways of describing movement are fundamental to movement analysis. You can use movement analysis to help you recognise your own idiosyncrasies and/or to note the movement capabilities of individuals with whom you are working, irrespective of whether this is one-on-one or in a group.[7]

Qualities drawn from movement analysis, combined with your knowledge of the individual needs and capabilities of any group, will help clarify movement aims and structure – effectively shaping the content of any movement session whether for your personal work or in work with others. In addition, it enables you to describe and record an individual's behaviour, your own, or that of a member of your group in simple movement terms, and to detail the changes that occur in your sessions over time.

Notes On Impulse(s) To Move (And Speak)

Movement initiated by an impulse involves the redistribution of weight (the body) in and through space:

- In moving this way, human beings create sculptures in and through space.
- Each shape is defined by:

    a +ve space (where the body *is*), and
    b -ve space (where the body is *not*).

The following points influence all human actions both on stage and in life:

- Movement comes from and returns to Stillness
- Sound comes from and returns to Silence
- All movement(s) and sound(s) involve energy:

    a Kinetic energy:

    - Intrinsic to the movement itself

    b Potential energy:

    - The impulse to move

        a The intention behind it

        - The Pause/Stop
        - Its importance to gathering energy for the next action(s).

When analysing movement, concepts, or events and/or when creating theatre, Jacques Lecoq suggested that our first task was to discover the 'essence', the bare bones framework of the matter. Lecoq always used an image – a fish skeleton – to illustrate his point. Once established, the framework can be 're-dressed' in chosen elements to reveal our message.

In the next section we look at some of the many reasons why daily movement is so important to health and wellbeing.

Notes

1 "[T]he ability to repeat a specific muscular movement with improved efficiency and accuracy that is acquired through practice and repetition." www.merriam-webster.com/dictionary/muscle%20memory
2 More than fifty years ago Ida Rolf suggested that the body is inherently a system of seamless networks of tissues rather than a collection of separate parts, something that the modern scientific study of fascia has validated. See https://blackroll.com/article/fascia-researchherently and www.rolf.org/rolfing.php
3 Later in this book we deal in more detail with how to prepare your body for action and thus prevent injuries.
4 This movement analysis is based on the principles of Rudolf Laban and adapted from a chart that originally appeared in 1981 as part of a teachers' pack (edited by C. Thomson and B. Warren) produced for LUDUS Dance in Education's programme 'The Thunder Tree' as part of their Learning Through Dance – Special Schools Project.
5 How We Move

Actions			*Qualities*		
Bounce	Pinch	Skip	Angular	Gentle	Thin
Carry	Pull	Slither	Bendy	Heavy	Weak
Catch	Punch	Stab	Curved	Hurrying	Wide
Crawl	Push	Stand	Dashing	Lingering	
Cut	Release	Step	Delicate	Long	
Fall	Rise	Stroke	Fat	Rounded	
Flutter	Rock	Tense	Firm	Short	
Hold	Roll	Throw	Flat	Small	
Hop	Run	Twizzle	Flickering	Spiky	
Kick	See-saw	Wave	Floating	Stiff	
Leap	Shake	Wiggle	Floppy	Tall	

Basic Descriptors

Body Parts (what you move)		*Directions (where you move)*		*Relationships (how or with whom)*	
Ankles	Knees	Backwards	Right	Against	Passing
Arms	Legs	Behind	Sideways	Containing/ Enclosing	Taking turns
Back	Mouth	Circle	Spiral	Contrasting	Together
Bottom	Neck	Down	Straight	Copying	With

Body Parts (what you move)		*Directions (where you move)*		*Relationships (how or with whom)*
Elbows	Nose	Forwards	Up	Following
Eyes	Shoulders	In	Zigzag	In groups
Feet	Toes	In front		In threes, fours …
Fingers	Tummy	Into the middle		In pairs
Hands	Whole body	Left		Joining
Head	Wrists	Out		Leading
Hips		Out to the side		Leaving

6 The irresistible joy of movement: for learning, exploring and leading into dance!
Here is a checklist guide to help identify strengths and weaknesses in themes in your assessment, in student improvement and overall enjoyment.

Elements Of Mvmt	*Directions For Locomotion*	*Levels*	*Physical Involvement*	*Tempos*	*Metaphors, Other Connections!*	*Kinetic Connections (adverbs)*	*Patterns*
				Fast forward	Hiccups	Slowly	Diagonal
Step	Forward	High		Reverse motion	Cough	Quickly	Straight
Lunge	Backward		Medium	Driving (aggressive)	Fast backward	Lava	Aggressively
Zigzag							
Skip	Fwd and back	Low	Stomping	Zoom-in	Sneeze	Smoothly	Circle in
Hop	Round and round			Zoom-out	Steam	Choppily	Circle out
Slide	Up			Freeze frame(s)	Maple seed falling	Lightly	Starburst
Turn	Down		Full body	Slow motion	Smoke		Spiral in
Twirl	Up and down		Arms only	Fade-in	Dandelion fuzz floating		Spiral out
Twist	Inward		Hands only	Fade-out	Evaporation		Wavy lines
Jump	Outward		Sitting		Gargling toothpaste		Concentric circles

Elements Of Mvmt	*Directions For Locomotion*	*Levels*	*Physical Involvement*	*Tempos*	*Metaphors, Other Connections!*	*Kinetic Connections (adverbs)*	*Patterns*
Glide	In and out		Torso only (no arms)		Condensation		Staggered lines
Tiptoe	Sideways		Torso and legs		Water/blood cycle		Continuous
Heel first	Side to side		Torso & arms		Popcorn		Broken (choppy)
Feet twisting	Crouch		On tummies		Volcano (steps of)		Random
Stomp	Curl		On backs		Lightning		
Pose	Stand		On sides		Metamorphosis		
Pause	Sit				Thunderclouds		
Roll	Crouch		Strength		Photosynthesis		
	Pivot		Agility		Boiling water, porridge		
	Jumble		Flexibility				
	Expand		Balance		Waterfall		
	Contract		Body-listening				
			Energy engagement		Bubbling brook		
			Focus				
			Concentration		Leaves in wind(s)		
					Water spiral (toilet)		
					Rain (various kinds)		
					Waves (various kinds)		

7 This can be especially helpful when working with individuals who have special needs. For example, which parts of their body, if any, can be moved in isolation? Can they balance with our aids? Can they travel? Can they travel, but only on the floor – that is, roll, crawl – or can they travel only in a wheelchair?

Chapter 3

Why Is Daily Movement So Important?

Every Movement Tells A Story

> One man in his time plays many parts,
> His acts being seven ages.
> (*As You Like It*, Act 2 Scene 7)

The longer one lives, the more stories we each have to tell about the life we have lived. Some stories are sad, some happy, some memorable, and others embarrassing. Many more are forgettable or not to be found within our memory but must be recounted to us by others who were there at the time the event happened.

During our lives we each experience minor bumps and bruises that limit our range of movement. Young children fall out of cribs or trees, or run into walls. As we grow older, we may experience bicycle, motorbike, or car accidents; slip on ice; twist our ankles, damage our knees or hips playing full contact sports; break collarbones diving for that spectacular catch. As older adults we fall off chairs reaching for cans high up in the cupboard; strain our backs gardening or lifting grandkids!

I (BW) throw myself into things, often quite literally! I have broken my collarbone, not once but twice! The first time I was about 17 teaching judo to a girl I really liked. I paid too much attention to her and not enough attention to what I was teaching! She threw me perfectly, I landed rather less so! I landed on the tip of my collarbone, very close to the left acromioclavicular (AC) joint, which I damaged and in addition cracked my clavicle! About 18 months later I outdid this when I launched myself at full stretch about shoulder height off the ground to execute a spectacular catch of a cricket ball. Unfortunately, not only did I hit the ground *very* hard, breaking my clavicle and damaging the AC joint on the *other* side, I also dropped the ball when I landed.

These are not my only major injuries. As a younger man, when I thought I was immortal, I damaged my knees, elbows, and neck through playing rugby and engaging in full contact martial arts. Later, while teaching theatre acrobatics, I fractured my spine (T10) through landing badly while performing a leaping diving breakfall when I had the flu! And I was dropped on my head

DOI: 10.4324/9780429439803-5

by students when demonstrating an inverted cross gymnastics move. I also injured my ankle performing a grand jeté over a snowbank in an icy car park in Montreal. Luckily, I finally twigged that I am not immortal and nowadays the most severe injury I experience is straining my shoulder joints carrying heavy bags from the grocery store.

The stories behind my injuries (GMF) are strangely the polar opposite of Bernie's – except when they are eerily the same. I have been fortunate – no broken bones. Like Bernie, my few serious strain injuries resulted from sudden actions, but unlike him, mine happened while I was alone, trying something someone else had 'told me about'. I was too impatient to wait for a teacher.

However, Bernie and I share eerily similar elements around spinal injuries. In my early twenties I 'fissured' three vertebrae in my neck and upper spine during a theatre acrobatics class. The teacher asked me to demonstrate a pairs-gymnastics move with a less experienced peer, who unexpectedly let go of me in mid-move. My head and neck were caught under my falling body. The injury was not helped by my catching a serious bout of 'flu' just afterward. I wore a neck brace for weeks, and the doctor advised, "No more headstands, ever!"

I recovered from the strain injuries, but as Bernie warns, they do come back to haunt us as occasionally recurring 'niggles'. As for my vertebrae – no headstands, and with mindfulness and gentle exercise, I can now keep my neck and shoulders free from tension, headaches, and pain. The great gift our bodies give us is that with care and attention, and unless there are extenuating circumstances, they can and do heal.

Importance Of Movement To Health And Wellbeing

In the late 20th and early 21st centuries people, especially those living in privileged countries, have become less active, more sedentary. This coupled with a diet of fast foods high in fats and sugar has led to a rise in obesity, heart disease, and type-2 diabetes and to the view that sitting has become, in terms of its effect on health, the new smoking. Job-related stress and the general pressures of balancing family and work have led to an increase in anxiety and other mental health conditions

More recently the Covid pandemic lockdown added another wrinkle in that many of us during lockdown experienced the double whammy of consoling ourselves with increased consumption of 'comfort' and 'junk' food and being inactive. Which amplified the problems already present in sedentary lifestyles that have, in large part, fuelled the modern obsession with fitness to compensate.

Observations During The Pandemic

I (GMF) moved into a 100-unit condo a few years before the onset of Covid. My seventh-floor unit overlooks the main entrance, visitor parking, and little garden area with numerous benches, and all units include a closed-circuit video of the lobby entrance. As watching people walk and move has been a lifelong obsession, I was perfectly placed to observe other tenants and their regular guests before and throughout this pandemic. Another opportunity was joining a varying group of tenants in bi-weekly 'fitness for seniors' classes, so I knew something of their pre-Covid physical and social behaviour. Then, Covid struck.

It has been shocking to see the effects of Covid on my fellow tenants, whether they were fitness class peers or simply people I 'knew' from continuous lobby/elevator/post office area encounters. While masking, distancing, and various degrees of lockdown have inevitably meant less-to-no socialising, it is the changes in physical mobility and appearance that have been most telling.

Formerly active and physically mobile tenants are slower, stooped, and nearly all of them have visibly deteriorated in terms of their ability to negotiate curbs, steps, or sidewalk irregularities, open doors, and get into and out of vehicles. I have observed a palpable and justifiable fear of falling off balance. They are slowly, but surely imploding into slower, more hesitant, awkward, and ever smaller 'cocoons' of themselves. Many of them walk with a limp, waddle, or shuffle. Backs are stooped and eyes are downcast. Many now need canes, walkers, or wheelchairs. Ambulances appear far more frequently. Many have left to live where they can get more care.

Simply put, the pandemic brought about a sea change in the movement capabilities of the residents I observed in my building. While these observations were not a rigorously conducted research project, they do seem to be in keeping with other anecdotal reports worldwide about the effects of inactivity and weight gain on overall health during the times of lockdown.

Chapter 4

The Benefits Of Movement

The health benefits of physical activity and exercise have been well documented. Extensive research shows a relationship between physical activity and not only reduced premature mortality but also the primary and secondary reduction of several chronic medical conditions. There are relationships between physical activity and health outcomes, and marked health benefits may be achieved with relatively minor volumes of physical activity.[1,2]

In addition, for more than thirty years research has shown that the benefits of physical activity for children are immense.[3,4,5] Incorporating movement throughout the school day makes students less fidgety and more focused on learning and may have both a physiological and developmental impact on children's brains.[6]

The findings of the research are simple: everyone can benefit from becoming more physically active – by regularly moving every day.

Some Well-Known Benefits Of Movement

There are so many benefits to be gained from moving every day.[7,8] The best known are:

- Increases blood flow and blood volume
- Cholesterol levels – lowers LDL, raises HDL
- Stimulates bone and muscle growth
- Weight management
- Lowers risk of heart disease, stroke, and cancer.[9,10]

A Few Other Benefits

Enhances Mood

Moving your body not only improves mood but also helps combat anxiety and depression. Movement increases the production of endorphins, which both act as a natural pain killer and help lift our mood. Endorphins are also

DOI: 10.4324/9780429439803-6

responsible for the famous 'runners high' and for making you feel relaxed and optimistic after a good workout.

One Polish study strongly suggests that exercise provides benefits both for healthy individuals for those with diagnosed emotional disorders, regardless of sex and age.[11] Other studies suggest that routine exercise, while not necessarily eliminating feelings of acute stress, is helpful in maintaining a positive mood and preventing stress from accumulating in your body.[12]

Improves Lymphatic System[13]

Unlike the circulatory or respiratory systems, the lymphatic system does not have a 'pump'. Instead, it relies on your motion to circulate lymph fluid around the body. Each time you move large muscles of the body, you help pump lymphatic fluid through your body, keeping your systems circulating. This enhances your immune response and overall health.

Aids Pain Management

Physical activity has benefits for people with arthritis. However, many people with arthritis do not exercise, often because of joint or muscle pain, weakness, fatigue, or joint swelling. This can lead to loss of joint motion, stiffness, and muscle weakness and tightness. These problems can worsen fatigue and can cause joints to become unstable.

There is a common misconception that exercise is deleterious to one's joints. However, it would appear that exercise has positive benefits for joint tissues in addition to its other health benefits.[14] Physical activity can decrease pain and enhance quality of life and is most beneficial when done on a regular basis.

Being physically active helps reduce inflammation, pain, and fatigue, and improves quality of sleep and mental health, which are all areas usually made worse by rheumatoid arthritis (RA). While being physically active is important for almost everyone, studies continue to show an even greater benefit for those with RA.[15]

Risks Of Physical Inactivity

At the same time as the weight of evidence argues for everyone engaging in daily physical activity, the problems associated with inactivity – most notably, simply sitting in one place for too long – have also been researched and highlighted.[16] The steady increase in childhood obesity and chronic illnesses associated with this is shocking.[17]

More recently, programmes to reverse this trend have been instigated. Many national and community-based sports and arts organisations have mounted programmes to encourage children to engage in regular physical activity. These seem to be having some positive effect.[18]

Notes

1 D. Warburton and S. Bredin (2017), www.ingentaconnect.com/content/wk/hco/2017/00000032/00000005/art00010
2 S. Baker (2021), www.thehealthhub.com/benefits-of-moving-everyday/
3 M.S. Southern et al. (1999), https://link.springer.com/article/10.1007/s004310051070
4 D.W Harsha and G.S Berenson (1995), www.sciencedirect.com/science/article/abs/pii/S000296291534979X
5 K.E. Powell (2019), https://journals.humankinetics.com/view/journals/jpah/16/1/article-p1.xml
6 D. Wilson and M. Conyers (2014), www.edutopia.org/blog/move-body-grow-brain-donna-wilson
7 CDC (2022), www.cdc.gov/physicalactivity/basics/pa-health/index.htm
8 R.R. Cosimo (2009), www.ncbi.nlm.nih.gov/pmc/articles/PMC2811354/
9 H. Zheng et al. (2009), https://pubmed.ncbi.nlm.nih.gov/19306107/
10 D. Warburton and S. Bredin (2006), www.ncbi.nlm.nih.gov/pmc/articles/PMC1402378/
11 M. Guszkowska (2004), https://europepmc.org/article/med/15518309
12 For example, see E. Childs and H. De Wit (2014), www.ncbi.nlm.nih.gov/pmc/articles/PMC4013452/
13 The lymphatic system is found throughout your body, removing waste from every cell while helping to regulate the immune system. It produces, stores, and transports white blood cells along a complex network of vessels, ducts, lymph nodes, the spleen, the thymus, the adenoids, and the tonsils.
14 D.J. Hunter and F. Eckstein (2009), www.ncbi.nlm.nih.gov/pmc/articles/PMC2667877/
15 P.J.W. Venables and K. Michaud (2022), www.uptodate.com/contents/rheumatoid-arthritis-treatment-beyond-the-basics
16 Hannah (2019), https://theheartfoundation.org/2019/08/10/is-sitting-the-new-smoking/
17 J. Wyszyńska et al. (2020), www.frontiersin.org/articles/10.3389/fped.2020.535705/full
18 W.J. Straus (2018), https://onlinelibrary.wiley.com/doi/full/10.1111/ijpo.12266

Part II

Space

In this section, the authors explore how space affects social performance and by extension the perceived and actual health of the individuals performing within it.

DOI: 10.4324/9780429439803-7

Chapter 5

Space And Eastern Philosophy

Taoist Views On Space, Energy And Health

For the Taoist, the universe is alive with a kind of primal power, a force they refer to as *Chi.*[1] Taoist belief suggests that not only do all living things possess Chi, we all live amid this vital force. Taoists believe, as do many physicists, that at the simplest level all life is pure energy.

One of the most important aspects of the Taoist conception of wellbeing is that to remain healthy we must constantly regulate our actions to remain balanced within ourselves and with the external and ever-changing universe. Taoist healers believe that the correct balance between Yin and Yang (opposite and complementary forces such as day and night, female and male) and the harmonious mixture of the five elements (Earth, Fire, Metal, Water, Air) makes for health: that the relative harmony of tendencies and forces within an individual *is* the individual's state of health. They contend that the opposite is also true, that lack of balance and disharmony cause disease.[2]

The process of identifying imbalances and re-establishing balance, both physically and emotionally, is one of the primary focuses of Taoist healing practice. In essence, Taoist healing seeks to strike a *double balance.*[3] Although the methods and concepts of practitioners vary, each healer, by utilising knowledge of the process, and their awareness of their own significance within that process, provides a framework for engaging each patient in a *dance towards wellness.*

Quantum physicists consider Chi a little differently. They suggest that a universal vital force (which the physicists conceive of as a field) exists always and everywhere and is the carrier of all material phenomena.[4] If they are correct, and we believe they are, then this has great significance for *any* space, whether it be personal, theatrical, social, or therapeutic.

Feng Shui, World Maps, and Performance Space

Successful human performance[5] in any situation requires an awareness of space and the rationale for actions to be performed in it. For several years I

DOI: 10.4324/9780429439803-8

(BW) was an actor/dancer in touring theatrical performances. During this time, I performed in a wide range of performance spaces – not only theatre stages but also pub courtyards, shopping malls, school gyms, and prison cafeteria. No matter where we were performing, I always walked the space before each performance *went up* to get a sense not only of the dimensions and acoustics of the space but also to get a feel of the energy within it. For the *Feng Shui*[6] of each space exerts an influence on each performance. For all spaces, even empty spaces, are alive and full of possibilities.

As Berger suggests, what we see situates us within our surrounding world. If asked we can describe and explain our world with words,[7] however as Korzybski pointed out the word is *not* the thing it describes.[8] So, even though we hear the sounds and feel the heat or cold and the energy of each space, irrespective of whether it is verdant landscapes of the countryside or the imposing architecture of a major city, we may not be able to adequately convey our responses to what we experience to another or others.

It should come as no surprise that Yogis and Qigong masters advocate performing Yoga and Qigong in natural surroundings. The therapeutic value to human health and quality of life of *green spaces* (e.g., woods, natural meadows, etc.) and *blue spaces* (e.g., rivers, seas, streams, canals, lakes, ponds, etc.), especially their inclusion within urban environments, is well documented.[9]

Spaces speak to each of us in different ways and create sensations within us as we respond to the energy and feel of each space. We have a visceral, a psycho-somatic, response to the space in which we exist. Yet how we each respond to any space is affected by what we each have experienced before we entered that space. Our genetics and our social upbringing and past social experiences are the lens through which we encounter and perceive each new space.

David Gordon expanded on neuro-linguistic programming theories to discuss how each of us creates, from a multitude of factors, a personal 'world map'[10] as a lens through which we interact with the stimuli we encounter in our day-to-day experience. Our world map is built upon our individual life experiences within the cultural matrices in which we experienced them. It gives each of us a sense of our place in the world. It provides the framework for our beliefs and prejudices but may be transformed with experiences over time.

Notes

1 Chi (also written as Qi, or Ch'i) has no direct translation in English. It is often translated simply as 'energy, but 'vital force', 'life force', or even 'creative force' more accurately describe it.
2 Veith (2002).
3 The double balance seeks to balance the energies of a body not only within, but also that the body must itself be in harmony with its surroundings, the space in which it exists.

4 Capra (1975).
5 For the purposes of this discussion, we define 'performance' as any action(s) taken by any individual or individuals within a space, for any reason,
6 Feng Shui, which literally translates as Wind-Water, is a traditional ancient Chines practice which considers the energies present in a space that help individuals be in balance within their surroundings (Fielding 2020).
7 Berger (1972).
8 Korzybski (1995).
9 Warren et al. (2019).
10 Gordon (1978).

Chapter 6

Theatrical Space

Entering An Empty Space

As Pendzik has suggested, 'Space' is that place where the invisible becomes visible.[1] It forms a barrier which must be crossed. And as Brook has suggested, the simple action, of crossing an 'empty space' with others watching is all that is necessary to begin the transformation of any space into a theatre stage.[2] This theatrical concept also applies to performance on a social stage, for when others are watching we change the way we behave.

Even if you do not think of yourself as an 'actor', human presence is all that is necessary for any room, any space to be transformed into a theatre – no special attributes are needed. It is also a liminal space[3] – a transition space, one you must cross over. Where you leave something behind, yet you are not yet somewhere or something else.

For example, when actors cross a space and engage the viewer in their performance, both the space and the viewers are transformed. The change from 'potential' to actual performer enacts a change not only on the viewer (from passive 'non-combatant' to active audience member) but also on the space (from geographic location to a 'theatre stage').

The Influence Of Bodies and Objects On Energy In A(ny) Space

Even a completely empty space is charged with possibility. It is full of energy. However, whatever or whoever inhabits the space affects the energy in the space and thus changes its flow and its architecture – its Feng Shui.

When a person walks across any space, anyone watching sees moving architecture. It is not simply that this movement transform this space into a performance space, it also reshapes the energy of that space. The person inhabits the space and in so doing they reshape the energy and the space itself. More than this they interact with it. Each item in the room has a relationship with the person walking through it. Any person moving across a space carves it into both positive and negative space. Identifying for viewers things that are there and things that are not.

DOI: 10.4324/9780429439803-9

The clothes that are worn move. The flow of the fabric influences the way an individual cuts the space, which shapes it into something architecturally different. The shape and colour evoke psychological responses in the viewer. All of which affects what any viewer sees and consequently how they react: how they feel about the performer moving across and sculpting the space.

Then there's the whole area of 'unexpected contradictions'. So often the walk, like the voice, can jarringly contradict what the viewer expected from their initial response to the individual's stature and costume, based on expectations drawn from their established world map. Watching an individual crossing a space, or speaking, for the first time may alter perceptions of who this stranger is. As the old saying goes, *you never have a second chance to make a first impression* – this is in a way the first line in an improvised story being created by the interactions between performer, viewer, and the space.

Feng Shui In Action: Architecture, Sculpture, and Performance

There is much to be learned about social performances from examining theatrical ones. As a director I (BW) always tried to sculpt space. When I directed, before it was seen by an audience, I always took time to sit and simply watch the play or dance unfold on stage. I tried to remind myself that the viewer did not attend the rehearsals and can only go by what they see on stage. So, I sat and watched the flow of movement and stillness and/or listened to words and silence in the way that I hoped the viewer would encounter them for the first time.

I was aware that not only did the set and lights, the movement of the performers but, as my colleague Professor Owen Klein often remarked, the words and speeches also have shape. Standing or moving on stage creates moving sculptures. The set creates architecture. The lighting and costume accentuate this. *All* create positive and negative space for those watching. Most importantly, it is the negative spaces (the emptiness) that defines what is present and enables the viewer to follow the action.

In 'The Kick', Barbara Morgan's photograph of the celebrated dancer and choreographer Martha Graham, Graham is wearing a long and voluminous dress. The dancer extends into space, yet holds her head downward, in an introspective, melancholic pose. While one leg extends in a curve outwards and towards the sky. This frozen, almost sculptural, image captures gesture, volume, and line, and shapes the space.[4,5]

Graham's renowned use of costume, colour, and lighting literally sculpts the space.[6] It momentarily freezes the full extent and journey of each movement, thereby expanding, filling in, and transmitting an increasingly powerful emotional and spiritual message that the viewer enters and experiences each second as it is danced. These observations from theatrical performance also speak to personal, social performances.

Notes

1 S. Pendzik (1994), www.sciencedirect.com/science/article/abs/pii/0197455694900345
2 Brook (1968).
3 The word 'liminal' comes from the Latin root, *limen,* which means 'threshold'. Seale (2016), https://transformationalpresence.org/alan-seale-blog/liminal-space-embracing-mystery-power-transition-will-2/
4 B. Morgan (1940), www.holdenluntz.com/artists/barbara-morgan/martha-graham-letter-to-the-world-kick/
5 www.gallery.ca/collection/artwork/martha-graham-letter-to-the-world-kick; https://www.youtube.com/watch?v=dYYs5P-ccS4
6 A. Kisselgoff (1984), www.nytimes.com/1984/02/19/magazine/martha-graham.html

Chapter 7

Interpersonal And Therapeutic Space

Creating A Safe Space Where Anything Can Happen

While Way advised drama educators that the drama room must be "a space where anything can happen",[1] in therapeutic work one must take this notion a little further. Here, it is not only a space where anything can happen, it also must also be a *safe* space, where the possibility exists to revisit traumatic events, memories, and emotions and to transform them and to reshape them through the power of drama. In doing so it may then become possible to tell a different narrative about our lives – a different, happier story about ourselves to tell others when we meet.

One of the reasons why the space must be safe is because within its boundaries participants transform into someone or something else, which carries the potential for revelation and/or significant personal meaning for all present in that space. While a dramatic moment, which carries the seeds of a real personal transformation, may happen in any theatrical performance, it is central to dramatherapy praxis. Consequently, within a therapeutic context it is crucial that the parameters of the space are delineated.

This sense of *a safe space where anything can happen* must start with and be reinforced by the leader of the session. For the leader helps the participants tell and reshape the narrative of their lives. This means both literally and metaphorically defining the emotional and physical limits to the space for the members of the group. This step is essential so that each individual participating feels comfortable enough to engage various aspects of self in the environment in which they are working.

Bridging The Space: Making Interpersonal Connections

Space exists between things and people. As Beckett suggests, we are born alone, astride of a grave,[2] and before we 'shuffle off this mortal coil'[3] our lives are spent trying to connect with others. To do this we must take risks and 'put our self out there'. We each must move, traverse the space, and bridge the gap between self and others.

DOI: 10.4324/9780429439803-10

Much of the time in our attempts to connect, to reach across the space, leaves us fumbling in the dark. Stumbling along trying to understand and read the rules of social interactions. Trying to reach across the space between self and others. Slowly learning to 'act normal'.

We grope and grasp at things and people and, if we are moderately successful, we learn to fit in. We find distractions, occupations, and people that enable to feel that we are a fully integrated member of the community in which our lives are enacted. If we do not manage to grasp the rules of social interaction necessary to integrate within our community then we stand out as socially incompetent or 'strange' – we are an outsider. One only must think how easy it is to know when someone is 'a tourist' in a new place. Even before speaking, they send off all sorts of nonverbal 'signals' that target them as 'other'.

Seeing The Space For What It Is

Sometimes we become trapped in the story we have created for and about ourselves but are oblivious to the energy and architecture of the space(s) in which we perform them. Often what we see is affected by where we look, and while familiarity often breeds contempt, it may also make individuals oblivious.

Over the years I (BW) have taught in many locations around the world. One exercise I often use to start a morning session is 'How I got here this morning'. This exercise asks each participant to briefly describe their journey from waking up in their bedroom to arriving at the classroom.

What I have found fascinating is not what people describe but what they do not. The sights and sounds on my journey to work, the street vendors, the bird songs, the landscapes, were new to me. Time and time again, I noticed things participants took for granted. This was especially true when I worked in Singapore, Shenzhen China, and the Gaza Strip. The participants were oblivious to the everyday sights and sounds of the location in which they lived.

This reminded me of a time when I was also guilty of this. Early in my career, when I worked in Shrewsbury, England, I encountered an architect who was also a historian with a special interest in medieval buildings. He made me aware that there are carvings and sculptures on top of many of the buildings which I had never been aware of because I was always focused on making my way to work quickly and efficiently – so, I never looked up.

Notes

1 Way (1967).
2 Beckett (1956).
3 Shakespeare (1603).

Chapter 8

Therapy And Performance In A Taoist Context

Chapter 8 looks at the interconnections between dance-movement performance, storytelling, and therapy within a Taoist context, going on to consider how 'creative moments' may help transform both inner personal and our performance spaces and enable us to 'dance towards wellness'.

Dance: Emotion In Motion

Recently I (GMF) was asked to help evaluate performances by young high school students enrolled in dance curriculum courses. The students had created and videoed their own performances. Due to Covid, some of these took place in school settings, while others were done in home locales. To level the playing field, all dancers wore masks, and all were videoed by a single camera in a constant position. There was one performance that stood out for me: a solo performed in what appeared to be the dancer's home that used the space and objects in fascinating ways.

The dramatic piece was a statement of the dancer's reaction to the pandemic. It was her story of her experiences told through movement. It started with the young dancer sitting at a very plain wooden table full of papers, with her head down on her hands on top of the papers. She stood up and slowly walked/danced around to the front of the table. From her dance sequences and technique, it was clear she was a novice dancer, but she was emotionally riveting. She ended up under the table, legs crossed and drawn up to her chest, arms around her knees and her head resting on her crossed arms. Somehow, she managed to transform that position under the table to represent a prison cell, a cave, and a refuge. It was simple, but compellingly powerful.

When she emerged, she transitioned into a very short series of simple pirouette-like turns and her arms went from an above-her-head dance position to a sudden break in form to shoulder height. As she turned, she bent over and instead of a pirouette, she swept all the papers off the table. The papers flew up and fanned out – an image of falling birds or thoughts or hope. It was a

DOI: 10.4324/9780429439803-11

visual image of despair. She slowly returned to her seated position behind the desk, head down in her hands once more.

Storytelling, Therapy, and Performance In A Taoist Context

In the above case, the dancer not only *tells* her story, she *is* the story: she has an intimate connection to and relationship with the space. Her interactions with the space help create a Taoist sense of balance for her. She communicates with her architectural surroundings and objects. The spotlight is on the performer, and because she is the resulting story, the viewer cannot help but feel and experience it deeply, as they accompanied her on her emotional, physical, and spiritual journey

Her dance illustrates and makes physical the Taoist idea of a *dance toward wellness.* It could be suggested that the table is an anchor in a sacred space. The table is, at first glance, the prison. The girl is trapped *at* it and *by* the papers. But she negotiates her own balance and wellness through her interactions with it as she transforms it into her 'safe space' by hiding under it.

Through her movements, gestures, and stillness – in tableaux-like poses or snapshot momentary 'stops' – she allows it to become a cave or 'security blanket'. There are fleeting times when we also see that the table she's hiding under for protection is also a prison cell, but it is through her energy that her transformation happens.

She isn't altogether free from the table and papers, but she emerges from under their yoke after sweeping the papers away. She still goes back to the table, and she'll have to deal with those papers, but she somehow now seems more 'in balance' with things. She has rejected, retreated, rebelled, and found some sort of reconciliation – and through her relationship with the table she is able to regain balance. Her relationship to the table is different at the end because she has, in her own way and time, come to terms with it – re-found her balance, her strength to continue, and interact with the task as a 'whole' person rather than being fully dominated by, submissive to, the table and those papers.

Creative Moments: Transforming Inner Space

Transformation is at the heart of any performance. Stage actors must transform from who they are in real life to who they are on the theatre stage. Similarly, social actors must transform by forging a blend of intellectual, emotional, physical, and spiritual energies into a single face, in theatrical terms, an appropriate mask which is then presented to others.

To perform appropriately we each must create the 'face' we believe we need to present. To do this we must assess the needs of each scene and make choices about how to enter each space and engage with the other people and objects within it.

To be successful social actors we need to be able to read the scene on which we are being expected to perform. Our ability to read the space. As already mentioned, this is affected by many factors. And if all of this wasn't enough, there is also the problem of 'irrational fears' *not* linked to a specific space or event – e.g., general anxiety, claustrophobia.

However, in the process of creating this new performance we become lost, if only momentarily, in a *creative moment* – a liminal state, itself a space between things, that possesses the potential to unite physical, intellectual, emotional, and spiritual aspects of our self. For in this momentary pause, when we are 'lost to the world', no matter how briefly, it is also possible that we may become open to change, and to opportunities for healing to take place.

Transforming Personal Space

Both the authors are privileged individuals. We live in what many would consider beautiful, open, airy, and well-appointed, tastefully decorated spaces with access to clean water, good lighting, heating/air conditioning, and a consistent power supply. Our living space, the 'where' of our personal story, is a positive 'character' in our personal narratives. This is not the case for everyone.

Many people live, if not in squalor, then in a less than salubrious living space. This space can exert a negative effect on mood and sense of wellbeing. During the pandemic many people became claustrophobic, overwhelmed, and depressed by not being able to leave their personal space. It severely affected the story they told about themselves. This reaction is not unfamiliar to many but pandemic *stay at home orders* amplified the feelings of ennui and alienation that many felt about their living space.

Not everyone has the capability to change the where of their story. And even if we do have the resources the move and subsequent transformation takes time. However, there are a few simple things that can, at least for a moment, change the energy of the space and our reactions to it.

- Create a 'focal point' in the space, something that draws one's eye – for example:
  a. A small light source in the room, such as a salt lamp or a table lamp with colourful shade;
  b. A picture or photograph of nature – water or open lands or mountains.

- Wear 'lively' clothes – for example:
  a. An outfit that has colours that make you feel good about yourself
  b. A 'cosplay' outfit you like – e.g., dress as:
     - Harley Quinn
     - Obi Wan Kenobi

  - Barbie
  - Hagrid.

- Wear comfortable clothes.
- Change your underwear to something that makes you feel good about yourself.

This dressing up and/or adding focal points or accents does not change the physical architecture of your living space. However, it can change its Feng Shui and/or your perceptions and reactions to it.

Part III

Staying Healthy In An Unhealthy World: Reframing Behaviours And Attitudes

In this section, in two short chapters the authors explore how our memories, previous behaviours, and experiences create self-imposed stress and impede our ability to live a healthy life.

DOI: 10.4324/9780429439803-12

Chapter 9

Mistakes And Bad Habits

How To Remove Them

Old Water Under Old Bridges: Avoiding Self-Imposed Stress

> No man ever steps in the same river twice, for it's not the same river and he's not the same man.[1]

We all carry memories around with us. Some we cherish and some we don't. They are the echoes of our story. Reminders of the steps we took along the path that has been our life. Some of these memories we cling to. They remind us of things we wish were still with us. We often long to return to the point in our lives that created the memory. We try to recreate the scene to travel back and relive the experiences. These are what I (BW) refer to as 'train journeys'. Here, a single moment from the past acts as a 'staging post' from which our mind takes a journey. It is as if we are sitting in a railway carriage looking out a window at the scenery the mind has created from past events.

Others come unbidden like a balloon bursting. These are usually strong memories hidden from conscious thought until triggered by a sensory stimulus – e.g., smell or music to which they were 'anchored'.[2] They may be overwhelmingly positive – e.g., those of our mother or of our first consensual kiss. Or they may haunt us, remind us of mistakes, of choices or actions we made that we wished we could take back or undo, or more traumatically remind us of things done to us without our consent.

Remembering past events, just like taking the occasional train trip, can be refreshing and *may* help us move forward to learn from our mistakes or build on our successes. However, no matter whether the memory is happy or sad, the times and events that created it have passed. For all our memories are like *old water flowing under old bridges.* The events that created them have already passed and can never be recreated.

None of us can live in the past. We may never go back, and nor should we for life demands we always move forward. If we do not find a way to prevent dwelling in our past, these recurring thoughts, even the good ones, can become our waking nightmares.

DOI: 10.4324/9780429439803-13

Obviously, our past experiences are all we have to negotiate the subtle and often confusing aspects of social interaction and our everyday life, but when we try to mould or bend each situation to our experience, rather than adapting to it as best we can, we cause ourselves stress, often sabotaging ourselves in the process.

Yet many people cause themselves unnecessary stress by trying to recreate moments from their past. Whether wistfully reflecting on perceived happiness as a child growing up or with one's own child, the brief moments of bliss shared with an ex, or success on the sports field, dwelling in the past for more than a fleeting few moments prevents us from focusing on the present and gets in our way. It can get to the point where trying to recreate past experiences creates stress for ourselves. We bring this into new relationships, whether at work or in our personal life.

Past experiences of this kind probably do not provide us with useful guidance on how to behave or react in the present. At this point we must let go of the past, focus on what is happening right now and develop new ways to adapt, or else we become socially disabled in the eyes of our peers and loved ones.[3]

The Way Of Doing Things: Relaxation, Intensity, And Incipient Stress

ESTRAGON: I tell you I wasn't doing anything.
VLADIMIR: Maybe not, but it is the way of doing it that counts, if you want to go on living.[4]

One of the major dichotomies of modern civilization is that individuals want to relax, but they can only allot short amounts of time to squeezing relaxing into their busy schedules. There was a cartoon in a Canadian medical journal that shows a patient asking the doctor how to relax. The doctor dutifully describes all the various ways of relaxing – meditation, mindfulness exercises, Tai Chi, Yoga, Qigong, and so on. To which the patient replies, "I'm learning how to relax, doctor – but I want to relax, harder and faster! I want to be on the cutting edge of relaxation".[5]

There are, to my mind, two types of stress: *situational stress* and *incipient stress.*

Situational stress tends to happen *to* us. There are a multitude of events that possess the potential to create situational stress. We are driving and someone cuts us off or we get involved in an accident; a person we love gets sick or dies; we are fired from our job.

To a large extent we must simply react to situational stress. We can employ simple techniques to calm our breathing and slow our heartbeat and pulse rate, and echo the Serenity Prayer by accepting the things we cannot change and focusing moment by moment on regaining control of those things we can.[6]

Incipient stress, on the other hand, we in large part create for ourselves. Gabor Mate refers to it as 'chronic daily stress'. Incipient stress begins early in our lives. It can become the sum of all unresolved issues and situational stress events encountered throughout our lives. Moreover, we are often not even aware of it. It is carried around on our backs like invisible clothing. This stress is "more insidious and more harmful in terms of (its) long-term biological consequences".[7]

I have a friend, let's call him Steve, who is a very successful business entrepreneur. For relaxation he goes dancing with his wife, practises Tai Chi and Qigong, and swims a lot. However, he tended to do everything in the same way he engages with his business – with relentless ferocity and intense drive. This approach is not always conducive to relaxation. As he grew older he started to develop various ailments, in large part due to his highly successful career as a competition martial artist during his youth, and because he had been in several automobile accidents.

Finally, he realized that he was suffering from incipient stress and a level of anxiety that he hadn't previously acknowledged. He realized he was engaging in everything, including his relaxation, in a way that was not good for his health. He made a vow to himself to slow down, to pause, to reduce the time at each activity and adopt a slower and more meditative pace. He has reduced the intensity and duration of his 'relaxing' pursuits, started to focus more on his breathing, and is already noticing a difference in his body.

Reframing Stress: What To Do With 'Found Time'

> There was a man who disliked seeing his footprints and his shadow. He decided to escape from them and began to run. But as he ran along, more footprints appeared, while his shadow easily kept up with him. Thinking he was going too slowly, he ran faster and faster without stopping, until he finally collapsed from exhaustion and died. If he had stood still, there would have been no footprints. If he had rested in the shade, his shadow would have disappeared.[8]

Today, time is always at a premium. Emails, texts, voice mails, phone calls, and meetings inundate us, to a point where it can take us most of our day just to keep up with correspondence. We often take work home with us. Many businesses are resource starved, and it seems that we are all being asked to do more with less. Constantly we are told we must 'work smarter, not harder', but what does this really mean?

Fear of not meeting deadlines and burying yourself in work, becoming a slave to your tasks, is neither the answer nor in your best interest. 'Beating yourself up' with unrealistic expectations and deadlines often builds up without our conscious knowledge and contributes to incipient stress, which as has already been discussed can be a silent killer.

A study in the *British Medical Journal*, which investigated job pressures and an employee's sense of job control, suggested that the effects of job stress are cumulative and may increase chances of coronary heart disease.[9] Moreover, a 2016 Conference Board of Canada report suggested that employees' stress-related problems cost Canadian business at least $32.3 billion a year.[10] Much of this stress can be prevented.

The stress we live with may be short term or chronic, but it is an inevitable and necessary part of life. Stress has a profound effect on the body's chemistry. During periods of stress the body produces chemicals that help us cope with the situation. However, these same chemicals may take their toll on the body, creating wild imbalances in metabolic function and sleep patterns, especially if these periods of situational stress are extreme or prolonged.

> When winds of change feel too strong
> close your eyes and let the breeze blow through hair.

Sometimes it is beyond our power to change the external factors necessary to alleviate our situation. Similarly, during periods of extreme duress it is exceptionally difficult to remove yourself from the source of the situational stress and we can often feel powerless. We are like a passenger on a jet dealing with pockets of turbulence while circling above a major airport waiting for clearance to land. In these situations, it seems that all we can do is sit back, finish our drink, look out the window, relax and enjoy the ride.

However, just as with the stresses of a long flight, there are some simple everyday things we can do to make the situation more comfortable:

- Drink sufficient clear fluids, especially water:
    - a Caffeinated drinks and alcohol both increase dehydration, and dehydration may magnify the negative effects of stress.
- Eat regular light and healthy meals.
- Most importantly, find ways to get sufficient rest:
    - a Deep sleep is one of the most restorative factors in dealing with both chronic and acutely stressful situations and helps the body's ability to repair itself.
    - b Short naps, especially in the afternoon, are also recuperative.[11,12]

Developing strategies and techniques to manage and reduce the effects of stress makes all the difference to whether we succumb to the pressure and become ill. Simply stepping back to identify the cause of the stress and implementing plans to change the situation will often be sufficient to resolve the problem.

A simple reframing of the situation may help to combat the frustration and stress arising from feeling rushed and out of control or overwhelmed. Rather than looking at time not involved in 'productive' activity as time wasted, why not view it as time *found*.

Surprisingly, finding time each day to simply *pause*. Get up from your desk and walk outside for two minutes helps break up your day. Afterwards, you will begin to feel more refreshed when you tackle the tasks required for the job.

Use your 'found time' to walk in a wood or sit and look at water. Practise Qigong or Yoga or any mindful meditation exercises – even a few minutes every other day will help transform your body, mind, and spirit.[13] A bonus is that some of these practices can be done *anywhere* – at your desk, in the car, while waiting in line at the bank or airport.

So, when next frustrated by waiting in line at the grocery store or bank, try not to take life so seriously. Realise that you have been given an unexpected gift – you have found time. A moment to rest, relax, and refresh yourself, mentally and physically.

Notes

1 Heraclitus, echoing Taoists sages who believed "you cannot step into the same stream twice".
2 First coined by William Twitmire, the term anchor(ing) is usually considered part of NLP. For more details, see www.nlpworld.co.uk/nlp-glossary/a/anchoring/
3 I (BW) explore this notion in detail in an earlier book, *Disability and Social Performance* (1988).
4 Samuel Beckett (1956).
5 Randy Glasbergen (2006).
6 Variation on the Serenity Prayer:
"God Grant me the serenity to accept the things I cannot change,
The Courage to change the things that I can, and the Wisdom to know the difference." https://en.wikipedia.org/wiki/Serenity_Prayer
7 Gabor Mate (2011). Mate also discusses these ideas in another excellent book, *Scattered Minds* (1999).
8 Chang-Tse. quoted in B. Hoff (1988).
9 H. Bosma et al. (1997), www.jstor.org/stable/25173847
10 www.newswire.ca/news-releases/unmet-mental-health-care-needs-costing-canadian-economy-billions-591988711.html
11 J. Li et al. (2016), https://agsjournals.onlinelibrary.wiley.com/doi/full/10.1111/jgs.14368
12 F. Dutheil et al. (2021), www.ncbi.nlm.nih.gov/pmc/articles/PMC8507757/
13 Throughout this book we provide suggestions, ideas and exercises that will help you to combat and avoid incipient stress.

Chapter 10

Mind Management

How we think affects how we act. Simple phrases and aphorisms can help us employ basic strategies to prepare for and ethically and successfully complete demanding tasks without undue stress or anxiety.

In India this approach is often referred to as 'mind management'.[1]

These simple phrases are signposts and guides – ways to manage impulses, thoughts, and actions to help achieve self-discipline. Attached to each are simple examples of activities, techniques, and practices that will enable you to slowly become more attuned to your own body, be aware of your place within the universe, and help with lifestyle choices and strategies that help combat stress and lead to a more healthful and happy life.

Life is Simple, But Not Always Easy

Life is simple – no matter what adversity we face we must accept the gift of life. Things, no matter how horrible and difficult they may be, happen for a reason, and as Nietzsche said, "What does not kill me makes me stronger". So – Smile, Breathe In, Breathe Out, Eat, Drink, Sleep. Repeat!

The past is past, and the future is yet to come … *this* moment is all there is. All that went before led to *this* moment; and *this* moment leads to all that follows. You may hope and plan for a future, but *now* is all there is. Focus on this moment *because* it is all there is. It is the only moment you may be sure of.

Understand Nature: Accept Your Place Within It

Tensions Between Water and Wood[2]

The image of water is always present in Qigong and Chinese martial arts.[3] This is an extension of Taoist philosophy, which talks of Tao as being a stream or a river. Taoist sages believe we are always immersed in Tao that our lives are spent in this moving river of life where we must surf its wave(s) – not only those of our own making but also of the universe we inhabit.

DOI: 10.4324/9780429439803-14

This is not always easy. We can surf in the same direction as the wave, or we can ride along it, but we *cannot* surf against its direction or else we are likely to 'fall off' our board. When this happens most of us simply pick ourselves up and get back on our surfboard, point it in the same direction as the wave, and continue our journey.

Root Like Tree ... Flow Like Water: Reflections on Yin and Yang

Sometimes a person need not teach for a willing student to learn.

In November 2011 I (BW) attended the Arts and Health conference held at the National Art Gallery Canberra, Australia. While there I met an amazing woman, Evelyna Yee. Known affectionately as 'grandma' she was an inspiration in so many ways. I listened to her speak, she took part in my workshops (co-taught with my late friend Dr Peter Spitzer), she and I talked a lot about the arts and health, and we shared a Qigong/Tai Chi session together in the Sculpture Garden: a fern garden with sculptures all around and a waterfall in the centre!

This experience was fantastic, moving in many senses of the word. Evelyna's movements were so fluid, and while I had seen many of the 'steps' before, because of her fluidity they were, for me, alien and at the same time transcendent and transformative. Watching her, and the few minutes we spent moving together, was an extraordinary experience. One that at the time was difficult to put into words: it was visceral, ephemeral ... it simply was!

A couple of days later back in Bowral at Peter's house where I was staying, I woke very early and started looking in detail at the pictures and short videos Peter had taken of Evelyna and I moving in the Fern Garden. As I looked, my first simplistic response was, my Chi is 'stale', solid, while Evelyna's Chi is 'alive', free. As I reflected a little more, I progressed to the thought that, as I am a man and Evelyna a woman, this was perhaps simply a Yang (masculine)/Yin (feminine) phenomenon. As it was still very early I went back to bed.

Later I got up to do my daily practice at sunrise outside on the balcony amongst the trees and kookaburras and lorikeets. As often happens during my early morning practice, my mind was nowhere in particular, and so it wandered. As I practised, my mind led me to reflect on Evelyna's comments about her affinity with water. In that moment it dawned on me: Evelyna's forms and practice are based on and influenced by water, while my regular Qigong exercises are based on Zhan Zhuang (standing like a tree): a form that helps to 'root me' and make me strong, but doesn't overly emphasise fluidity and flexibility.

Comparing oneself to anyone else is always fraught with problems. However, it is not that I do not flow or that I lack fluidity, it is simply that to my eye Evelyna is like a stream, her every gesture flowing effortlessly from the one before. So out there on the deck miles from home as the sun rose in Australia, I tried something different in my usual set of exercises. I started to see if I could add fluidity to my forms. Trying to remain true to the notion of 'do without doing' while at the same time making my Chi dance.

I started by focusing my energy, allowing Yi (mind) to lead Chi (energy). I was trying to add water to my tree. As I slowly let go of conscious thought it was a revelation! My body was allowing Chi to flow. I was flowing between stability and motion between Yin and Yang. My motions and forms while similar felt lighter, more alive, and less measured.

The point of this long anecdote is that even after more than forty years of study with some of the best teachers one could ask for, it is always possible to learn more and to move further along the path. There are no coincidences. I did not expect a chance meeting at an arts conference to take my forms and practice to another level. Evelyna was not my teacher; she is by her own admission "not a Chi master" and maintains that she still has "much to learn". Yet at that moment I was ready, willing, and able to listen to the universe and to learn from whatever it presented.

Notes

1 In Taoism this is often referred to as Yi(yee) leading Chi(chee) – thought directing energy.

2 B. Warren et al. (2018), https://juniperpublishers.com/jcmah/pdf/JCMAH.MS.ID.555673.pdf

3 Martial artists are always trying to find a balance in the 'tension between rooting like a tree and flowing like water' – that sense of being both rooted and flowing. It is a 'wood', but they must strive not to become wooden. Whereas female martial artists are water, and they must strive to find roots.

Part IV

Simple Ways To Re-Integrate Healthy Movement Into Your Daily Life

In this section the authors present ways to pursue a personal routine in small spaces in your own home using Qigong and Yoga. The information shared is based on data collected from extensive research and personal praxis over fifty years.

The authors suggest there is no need to purchase expensive gym memberships, which are often not used. The section provides clear directions on how to begin an Eastern-based movement exercise programme at home and outlines some of the values of such practice to personal health.

DOI: 10.4324/9780429439803-15

Chapter 11

No Need To Go To A Gym

Exercising In Small Spaces At Home

The road to hell is paved with good intentions.[1]

Many people spend a lot of money each month on gym and health club membership. These memberships go up after Christmas and New Year as individuals make resolutions to get in shape and lose weight. Unfortunately, many do not carry through with their resolutions.[2]

The reality is that although gyms, athletic clubs, and studios, with their diverse programmes and personal trainers, offer many options and opportunities for health and fitness, it is not necessary to attend them to get healthy. You do not have to block out 30–90 minutes or walk, cycle, or drive down to the gym to get healthy. It is possible to pursue life and health goals through a personal routine in your own home using Qigong[3,4] and Yoga[5,6,7]-based exercises – each of which has a documented history dating back more than 3,000 years.

Modern research has shown the benefits from pursuing such low-impact and low-risk Eastern-based programmes not only for persons with medical conditions (e.g., cancer; cardiac and respiratory problems; high blood pressure, diabetes, arthritis, and even spinal cord injuries[8]) but also for relatively healthy individuals seeking to prevent illness, reduce stress, anxiety, and depression, manage pain, sustain an active lifestyle, and increase longevity[9,10].

No Time (Or Space) To Practice? No Excuses!

Excuses are plentiful and cheap. We have all found reasons why we cannot do something. However, the beauty of the exercises presented here is that they can be done almost anywhere, at any time, and at no cost.

It is possible to do most Qigong and Yoga exercises in very limited space. Qigong can be done seated, standing, or moving and provides a thorough, non-stressful, and extremely low-impact work-out for the whole body. It requires no special or expensive equipment. Yoga can be done using a mat, a wall kitchen counter, or sink.

DOI: 10.4324/9780429439803-16

Where Should I Practice?

The standing exercises presented here can be done almost anywhere. Many of the more sedentary exercises e.g., *Standing Like A Tree*, are subtle enough that they can be performed while waiting for a bus or standing in line (at the bank, a grocery store, etc.), or at home.

Every day, I (BW) use different sets and combinations of these Qigong and Yoga exercises at home in my small apartment in 2–3-day rotations. This allows me to cross train my body, working different sets of muscles and strengthening different physiological and immunological facets of my body.

Preparing Your Home for Practice

Here are some simple guidelines concerning where, when, and how to practice the exercises that follow.

An ideal space is one that is quiet and open and with good light and a view of trees and/or water. However, if this is not available find the most tranquil space and view available to you.

Preparing The Room

Try to create a clean quiet area, one that provides:

- Minimal distractions – if you live in a city apartment on a busy road, try to find the quietest space possible.
- Move back furniture to create as large an open space as possible.
- Even on the coldest winter day it is important to open a window(s) to let in fresh air.
- Sweep, vacuum, or mop the floor regularly.
- If using counters or sinks for stability, clean and dry the surfaces.
- If there is a fan in the room, turn it on low.
- Close heating vents and/or turn down the thermostat.

As electricity can affect the flow of Chi, try to practice away from electrical cables and overhead power lines. Even being too close to a wall carrying electrical wires may disrupt the flow of Chi.

Preparing Your Body

Many ancient texts have very specific directions about preparing the body for practice. These can include such things as cleansing the mind and the nine openings of the body. However, for most of us, trying to find time to do this before we engage in exercise to help us cope with daily life is likely to increase rather than reduce our stress!

Simply rushing from a stress-filled work or home and expecting to instantly benefit from the exercises presented is a tall order. So, before you begin, simply take three long, slow breaths, letting go of your thoughts and troubles on each out-breath.

What Should I Wear?

It is possible to practice in any outfit (or even naked); however, it is probably best to wear loose comfortable clothes. For example:

- T-shirt and/or sweatshirt
- Yoga, 'harem' or track pants.

I would also recommend wearing:

- Layers, so that you can add or remove clothing as needed
- Breathable and natural fabrics.

It is best to remove as much jewellery as possible as it can affect the flow of energy. This includes your watch, bracelets, and earrings, as well as any other body-piercing rings.

When practising indoors at home, being barefoot or wearing light cotton socks works well. If you feel the need to wear footwear, then wear a light shoe, like water shoes or canvas deck shoes or martial arts slippers. Try to avoid heavy runners or cross trainers as they often restrict energy flow through the ankles.

When Should I Practice?

I am often asked what time of day is best to do practice? While Ancient texts often have very specific directions about when to practice, what direction to face, what exercises should be done, what time to gain maximum benefit,[14] I usually suggest that there are four times of day that are particularly good: sunrise, midday, sunset, midnight. However, after that I usually recommend choosing any time you can find that will work for you consistently!

How Often And For How Long Should I Practice?

My suggestion is always to start slowly and build up. At the beginning if you can build these exercises into your routine 2–3 times a week that is a good start.

Many people like to create a routine, a time they set aside to practise these exercises. Others fit in the exercises wherever and whenever they can. Finding even 5–10 minutes at any time during the day can produce positive effects.

Like most exercise programmes, the effects of the exercises in this book are cumulative. Initially it is better to do a two-minute *burst* twenty times during the day than forty minutes all at once. As your body becomes more accustomed to these exercises you can extend the time you allocate to your practice! One simple way to do this is simply to increase the number of repetitions for each exercise or set of exercises.

Also remember that you do not need to do any single exercise or set of exercises obsessively. Like cross training, varying your choice of exercise(s) is not only a good idea, in the long run it is better for you.

Should I Play Music While Practising?

I am often asked about whether to use music. This is, I feel, very much a personal choice. Like many other people, I often play soft relaxing music while I practise (even when I am outside), especially when teaching classes. However, I know many teachers and practitioners who prefer silence or natural sounds when outside.

In the last several years the availability of New Age music has led to a wide range of possibilities. Currently I use:

- Deuter: *Wind and Mountain* – particularly the tracks 'Wind and Mountain' and 'Island in the Sun'
- Yatao: 'When The Wind Talks'
- Parijat: *Buddha Garden* – particularly 'Raindance.

However, over the years I have also used various other pieces of music – for example:

- Pachelbel: *Canon in D with Ocean Waves*
- Anzan: *Reflections of Nature: Zen & The Art of Relaxation.*

Notes

1 The saying is often attributed to Saint Bernard of Clairvaux, although others suggest its origin is much earlier, being a paraphrase of a quote in Virgil's *Aeneid.*

2 Recent research (2018 n=4,000) found that 95% of New Year's resolutions are fitness related; it also found that 43% of people give up their goal after just one month, and after just three months, only 10% of people had stuck to their fitness resolution.

3 Qigong (usually translated as breath power or energy work), the Chinese practice of aligning breath, movement, and awareness for exercise, healing, and martial arts training, extends back more than 4,000 years.

4 According to the traditional Chinese medical community, the origin of Qigong is commonly attributed to the legendary Yellow Emperor (2696–2598 BCE) and the classic Huangdi Neijing book of internal medicine.

5 The beginnings of Yoga were developed by the Indus-Sarasvati civilization in Northern India around 2700 BCE.

6 Yoga is more than the physical asanas associated with modern Yoga classes. The true meaning of Yoga is union with the Divine. The *āsana*, or bodily stretching, is a relatively new phenomenon that has arisen in the last century.

In pre-modern India, the *āsana* was always *one auxiliary among many* of a complete psycho-physiological system of disciplined Yoga practice, enjoined alongside other Yoga directives including: ethical restraints and observances (*yama* and *niyama*), breath control (*prāṇāyāma*) and retention (*kumbhaka*), bodily seals (*mudrā*) and binds (*bandha*), and meditation techniques (*dhyāna*).

7 S. Ezrin (2021), www.healthline.com/nutrition/13-benefits-of-yoga

8 Even more profound is the use of Qigong in combination with modern Western medical approaches.

9 R. Jahnke et al. (2011), www.ncbi.nlm.nih.gov/pmc/articles/PMC3085832/

10 B. Frantzis (2011), www.energyarts.com/qigong-benefits/

Chapter 12

Starting Simply

Basic Tips For Safe Daily Movement Practice

- *Breathe with the movement*

  a Breathing with the movement, especially synchronising your breathing with your movement, greatly reduces the chances of pulling, straining, spraining, tearing, or breaking ligaments, tendons, muscles, bones, etc. This applies to all forms of movement, including:

  - In ballet, a lift in a pas de deux, or a grand jeté
  - In basketball, a jump shot.

  b Always exhale 'on the effort'.
  c *Never* hold your breath or breathe against the movement.[1]
  d Breathe from your diaphragm, not just the top of your lungs.
  e *NB If you have a heart condition or circulation problem*, do *not* hold your breath or 'suck in' stomach muscles (especially while breathing in).

- *Keep your knees and hips relaxed*

  a Do not 'lock' or hyper-extend your knees.
  b When bending your knees, be sure never to extend them beyond the end of your big toes.
  c Your knee should point in the same direction as your 2nd toe (next to big toe).
  d *NB Keeping your knees supple helps prevent heart attacks*

  - Many nerves, blood vessels, and meridians run through your knees
  - Keeping your knees moving allows the heart to pump blood more efficiently.

- Unless stated otherwise in the text follow this pattern:

  a *When moving your arm(s)*

  - As your arm(s) rise – breathe *in*
  - As your arm(s) lower – breathe *out.*

DOI: 10.4324/9780429439803-17

b *When moving your leg(s)*

- As you raise leg(s) – breathe *in*
- As you lower your leg(s) – breathe *out.*

Some additional comments:

- Any sharp pains are a sign from the body to stop/slow down or readjust your position.
- Warmth and/or tingling is a sign that Chi is flowing through the body's meridians.
- You may also see your palms grow red – a sign of blood flow through to the extremities.
- The way you breathe influences the functions of the body:

  a Qigong breathing patterns help to improve the immune and lymphatic systems and aid digestion
  b Done correctly, they also improve oxygen uptake and all movements.

- *Relaxed tension* – use the minimal amount of energy to hold yourself up and in place.
- 'The legs are the second heart' – modern research has echoed this sentiment, arguing that keeping them strong helps with the pumping of blood and thus the prevention of strokes and heart disease.
- If you *take care of your own body* you will have a greater chance of preventing illness through stress.

East Meets West Approach To Exercise

Several years ago, I (BW) injured my hip. The issue was in part age related, but mainly it was aggravated from sitting and driving fifty kilometres each way to work every day. I also had (and still have periodically) problems with both knees, injuries sustained from playing full contact sports (when I thought I was immortal) and extremely tight IT bands, which exacerbated the problem. Over the years, I tried chiropractic and massage (at the time I had a wonderful chiropractor and a marvellous massage therapist), and these treatments did help for a while, but the problem always returned.

I decided to see a physiotherapist. At the time she was hosting my Qigong classes at her clinic and was also one of the Qigong students. While we always had heated discussions about East and West approaches to healing, we respected and learned from one another and from time to time simply agreed to disagree!

I first saw her for about six weeks.[2] After each session she always sent me home with a set of exercises which I often adapted, based on my own knowledge. Anyway, many of my homework tasks were adapted Yoga exercises.[3] These helped reconnect me to the Yoga I had studied several years before.

Since that first visit, I have included therapeutic Yoga exercises in my weekly routines, and I now try to practise these 3–4 times a week. As a result, my daily practice now takes a lot longer. It includes rotating daily Qigong/martial arts sets[4] (25–40 mins) and floor wall and counter stretches (15–20 mins) as well as swimming (5–10 mins) when I have access to a pool.[5]

All the sets I practise include mindfulness and meditation. Some days, I do not feel like doing a full set, and on these days I do a shorter session – but I make sure I do some home-based exercises at least five days a week.[6]

(Almost) No Time Or Space Required

Many of the exercises require little or no preparation and can be performed almost anywhere, at any time, for as long or as briefly as you like. All you need is enough room to raise each arm out in an arc from your sides to above your head and a little clear wall area. Or space to place a mat or blanket on the floor. The health and energy benefits of simply doing even five minutes of these exercises two or three times a week will start to show within 4–6 weeks. A full description of these exercises appear later in the book.

Wall And Floor-Based Adapted Yoga

As already mentioned, I have a series of adapted Yoga exercises that I perform 3–4 times a week to help combat the various injuries mentioned above. These injuries have been aggravated by a genetic predisposition to knee problems that runs in my family and the weight I have gained since I turned fifty. I have found that even five extra pounds (2.2 kgs) aggravates my problems. While an extra ten pounds (4.5 kg) creates the possibility of being confined to bed. So, I watch what I eat and try to keep my weight within a manageable target range for health reasons, *not* because of vanity. I should add two caveats: I am not always successful in this goal and I, like most people, do care what I look like!

Wall-based exercises I do regularly in sequence are variations on/modified versions of:

- Stirrup/Happy Baby Pose (Ananda Balasana)
- Legs Up The Wall Pose (Viparita Karani)
- Butterfly Dries Its Wings (Titli Asana)
- Reverse Pidgeon/Eye Of The Needle Pose (Sucirandhasana).

The floor-based exercises I do regularly are variations on/modified versions of:

- Corpse Pose (Savasana)
- Eye Of The Needle with Spinal Twist
- Lying Butterfly Pose/Reclining Bound Angle Pose (Supta Baddha Konasana)
- Reclined Spinal Twist (Supta Matsyendrasana)
- Floor Sun Salutation Child Pose (Balasana).

Exercising While Standing At The Kitchen Counter[7]

For over forty years I taught dance-movement classes to students and professional artists of all ages and abilities. In 1984, I came across the marvellous book, *Teaching Dance to Senior Adults*, by the wonderful Liz Lerman. What I read and saw of her work was an inspiration. One thing that stuck in my mind was her use of chairs, instead of the traditional stationary handrail, for barre work – ballet and dance training and warm-up exercises. Now thirty years later I find myself using my kitchen counter and bathroom sink for barre work and some Yoga exercises.

Counter work exercises I do regularly are variations on/modifications of Yoga:

- Plank Pose (Phalakasana)
- Cobra Pose (Bhujangasana).

I also do a very simple exercise at my kitchen counter which is a combination of ballet barre exercises, Kung Fu/Qigong (Flying Crane) and Yoga (Virahandrasana III/Warrior Pose III), which I call 'ballet meets martial arts'.

Free-Standing Exercises

Zhan Zhuan – Standing Like A Tree

In strict traditional martial arts practice novice students are often required to hold individual postures for long periods of time and must 'master' the architecture of the pose before learning the next. This standing practice is an essential part of the traditional martial arts practice and has many benefits.

For the martial artist, it helps the body remember the exact position of a block or strike so that, like driving a car, when a move is needed it is instinctual.

More than this, when holding a posture without effort, blood and energy flow more freely, helping to strengthen the body and bring all bodily functions into balance.

Yi Chuan/Zhan Zhuang: Simple Energy Circle

Unlike Western-influenced exercises, where participants are constantly moving, standing still, and holding a single posture for long periods of time is a hallmark of Eastern-influenced exercise.

An energy circle is a sequence of standing postures that are ideally held for eight slow breaths,[8] and follow a pattern that begins and ends at the same point. The simple sequence of postures presented in this book can be done almost anywhere.

Notes

1 There are exceptions to this rule – e.g., in the dance performances of Martha Graham, where working against the breath was an emotional statement.
2 Over the next ten years I visited periodically when I experienced other minor structural issues with my body.
3 These exercises were drawn from P. Egoscue and R. Gittines (2000), *Pain Free: A Revolutionary Method for Stopping Chronic Pain* (New York: Random House) and S. Powers (2008), *Insight Yoga: An Innovative Synthesis of Traditional Yoga, Meditation, and Eastern Approaches to Healing and Well-Being* (Boulder, CO: Shambhala Publications).
4 A set is a series of exercises done in a particular sequence – e.g., the Ba Duan Jin. A set may also include several sets of exercises also done in a particular sequence.
5 I have access to an outdoor pool at my building from May until October. Also, I swim when I am away from Canada in the winter, usually December–March.
6 At the time of writing I am almost seventy years old and have been practising Eastern-based exercises for nearly 55 years.
7 These exercises can also be performed on the balcony of a ship or an apartment (flat). Simply use the railing instead of a kitchen counter.
8 Each of the postures presented may be held for as few as three breaths or as long as you feel comfortable. I usually hold each posture for eight long, slow, unhurried breaths. Master Lam (1991) recommends building up to twenty minutes for each posture.

Part V

Essential Eastern Exercises

In this section the authors build on ideas introduced in section IV. Each chapter describes in detail specific exercises to help reduce stress, promote health, and prevent illness drawn primarily from the Eastern health practices of Qigong and Yoga.

DOI: 10.4324/9780429439803-18

Chapter 13

Walking The Silk Road: Essential Eastern Exercises

Essential Standing Exercises

There are three basic standing exercises described in this book:

- Standing Like A Tree
- Standing Post
- Inverted Y.

Standing Like A Tree

Standing Like A Tree is a self-healing exercise, and the de facto basic standing exercise for all stationary Qigong. It is considered one of the so-called 'Great Medical Treasures' of classical Qigong. It is a simple but potent weapon in the fight against stress and stress-related diseases. Moreover, research suggests that standing for five minutes in this position has the same cardio-vascular effect as walking for twenty minutes on a treadmill at a moderate pace. This posture can be done while waiting for a bus or in a line up, before or after doing the dishes, or anywhere where you are standing!

- Stand with your legs hip width apart and your feet flat on the floor parallel to one another.
- Bend your knees but do not let them extend beyond your toes.
- Keep your shoulders relaxed and your spine straight *but not rigid*.
- Imagine that your head is suspended from the sky by a silken thread, that there is a small cushion of air between each vertebra, and that your chin rests on a silken pillow, so that your eyes remain parallel to the floor
- Move your hips slightly backwards, as if sitting down on a high bar stool, so that your shoulders are slightly forward of your hips.
- Point your elbows away from your body with your palms facing towards your thighs.
- Do *not* tighten your stomach muscles – rather, keep the front of your body soft.

DOI: 10.4324/9780429439803-19

- Throughout this exercise think of your head 'floating up' and your tail-bone 'drifting down'.
- When properly aligned you should feel a gentle stretching sensation in your inner thighs and buttocks.
- *You should imagine that you are like a tree*, rooted to the ground through your legs and feet, reaching upward to the sky through the top of your head.
- In the beginning hold this position for about 30–45 seconds. As you become more comfortable with the position you can slowly increase your time in this position until you can stand like a tree for five minutes.

Standing Post

- Stand with your feet together, big toes touching, and keeping your:

  a Legs straight with your knees relaxed and not locked
  b Eyes parallel to the ground
  c Arms held loosely by the side of the body with palms facing your thighs
  d Spine straight but not rigid.

Tips:

- Focus your eyes on a point in the distance.
- If practising outside choose a tree or a tall building or the horizon.
- Keep your shoulders relaxed and the front of your body relaxed.

Precautions: keep your knees relaxed – do *not* lock knees.

The Inverted Y Position

The *Inverted Y* position links directly to traditional Chinese calligraphy. The symbol for a human being was often an inverted Y shape with a straight line drawn across at the junction of the 'V' and the 'I' to represent the arms. As a result, this position is sometimes referred to as the 'Mankind' or 'Human Being' posture. Unlike the *Standing Like A Tree* position, you must keep your knees straight but again *not* locked. Initially this can be more difficult to achieve than it seems.

- Stand with your:

  a Legs shoulder-width apart – approximately one foot and one fist width between the arches of your two feet
  b Feet flat on the floor, parallel to one another
  c Knees straight, but not locked

d Shoulders relaxed
e Spine *straight, but not rigid*
f Your eyes looking at a point in the distance that is parallel to the ground.

Breathe And Smile: Notes On Breathing And Health

Once you have practised the basic standing exercises without worrying about how and when to breathe, it is time to focus on your breathing as if your life depended on it.

Heart Of The Breath: Finding Dan Tien

In Eastern texts the Dan Tien is often referred to as the seat of the breath and/or the wellspring of Chi. Dan Tien (pronounced Dan Tee-en) is described as being located about two inches below the body's surface at a point approximately three fingers below the navel.

In addition to the style of breathing known as *natural breathing*, there are many other styles of breathing employed in the Chinese tradition of martial arts – e.g., *reverse or Taoist breathing*, where the abdomen moves outwards on the out breath and inwards on the in breath.

The breath itself can be:

- *Cleansing* (in-breath is through the nose and out-breath is through the mouth)
- *Relaxing* (out-breath is longer than the in-breath)
- *Enervating* (in-breath is longer than the out-breath), or
- *Healing* (in-breath is directed to a point of tension or pain and the pain is expelled on the out-breath).

Natural Breathing

- Focus on your breathing

 a Breathe *in* – Clear Your Mind
 b Breathe *out* – Cleanse Your Body.

- Try to breathe in *and* out through your nose –
- Slow, natural, regular breaths

 a Keep your mouth closed
 b Your teeth gently touching
 c Tip of your tongue gently touching the roof of the mouth
 d *Above all, do not hold your breath.*

- Breathe through your nose with the tip of the tongue touching where teeth touch upper palate – breathe naturally. In your mind's eye:

  a Imagine the oxygen you are breathing in is a coloured gas
  b Visualise this gas as it enters the body into your lungs.

- Form a heart shape around your belly button by placing your thumbs above your belly button and the tips of your fingers on the pubic bone.
- Breathe in through the nose down to the heart-shaped area.
- Feel hands move away from body (stomach area) as you breathe in – breath in = belly goes out.
- Keep your feet parallel, teeth lightly touching, lips softly closed, tongue resting on top of the palate close to the teeth.
- Allow tension to 'relax out' as you breath out.
- Hands often start to tingle or shake (if they do not, there may be tension which cuts energy flow – release your joints by relaxing elbows, shoulders, wrists, fingers)

  a Fingers should be open, as if there were tiny little marbles in between them.

- Remember, always try to *synchronise your movements to your breathing.*

Finding The Heart Of The Breath

- Stand in the *Standing Like A Tree* pose.
- Form a heart shape between your two hands by

  a Placing your hands palm down on your belly, your thumbs almost touching, the tips of your fingers resting on/pointing towards your pubic bone, thus forming a heart shaped area around your navel.
  b This locates the position of the Dan Tien – 'the heart of the breath'.

- Close your mouth and half close your eyes.
- Breathe in and out through your nose.
- Guide air into the 'heart' area.
- Breathe slowly and smoothly, with as little effort as possible.
- Once you have located the Dan Tien and are able to breath regularly into this point, let your arms relax by your side.
- The breathing pattern described in heart of the breath is the one used in all exercises in this book, unless stated otherwise.

Tips:

- Try to keep your breathing as regular as possible

- It is helpful to imagine the breath as a column of air or a stream of water
- Try to regain the softness of a baby's breath
- *Do not be afraid to let your mind wander.*

Benefits:

- Helps collect and store energy
- Helps regulate heartbeat and calm anxiety.

Opening And Closing Breaths

I (BW) begin my daily Qigong practice with a physical clearing and cleansing using a set of three linked exercises which together are known as the *Opening and Closing Breaths.* These exercises help to 'guide' Chi through the main meridians, energise the body, and expel 'stale' air.

This set of exercises is also referred to as the *Three Healing Breaths* because they help to strengthen the immune system and cleanse the body of impurities and, in Traditional Chinese medical practice, are used to help prevent and treat cancers and stress-related diseases.

They are best performed at the beginning and/or the end of every session.

- Ideally, breathe *in* and breathe *out* through your nose where indicated below, or simply breathe naturally without holding or forcing your breath
- Repeat each exercise three or more times up to a maximum of eight, then proceed to the next.

Begin all three by assuming the *Standing Like A Tree* posture.

Lotus Flower Opening

- Breathe *in* – open your elbows sideways so that your hands lift away from floor palms up towards the sky.
- At your navel turn palms down, pointing your fingers towards the ground.
- Slowly lift your hands above your head … until your fingers point towards the top of your head.
- Open your hands outwards … your palms towards the sky.
- When your hands reach shoulder height breathe *out*, turning your palms down towards the ground.
- Continue until your arms are at your side.

Lotus Flower Closing

- Breathe *in* – open your arms sideways as if a large balloon is inflating.
- At heart height, turn your palms towards the sky.

- Lift your arms in an upward circular motion until your palms face the top of your head.
- Bring your elbows together so that they face forward
- *Breathe out* – slowly move your elbows towards floor with your palms facing your body and your fingers pointing towards the sky.
- At navel height, open your elbows sideways, move your hands towards the ground
- Continue until your arms are at side.

Petals Floating On The Water

- Raise your hands to navel height, turning them until your palms face towards your navel.
- Breathe *in* – float your elbows sideways, your palms following the motion of your elbows.
- Breathe *out* – begin to bring your elbows towards body with your palms following the motion of your elbows.
- At end of exercise cover your navel, one palm on top of the other. Breathe naturally.

Essential Postural Exercises

The Celestial Stem

Celestial Stem is a term used to describe how the spine should be 'held' with each vertebra aligned one on top of the other and the space between each vertebra equidistant.

The Celestial Stem describes the point from the top of the spine (inside back of the head that points to the sky) to the tip of the tailbone. This needs to work as a single unit and keep aligned – if it curves or twists to one side, this blocks blood flow and impedes free movement.

- Paying attention to the Celestial Stem helps:
- With general day-to-day movement
- Protect the lower spine
- Alleviate abdominal and menstrual cramps
- With digestion and weight and body changes.

To achieve this:

- Imagine a string attached to the top of your head that lightly and softly pulls you up to the sky.
- At the same time, imagine a string is attached to your tailbone that lightly and softly pulls your tailbone down to the floor.

- Maintain 'relaxed tension' – that is, keep:

  a Your shoulders, chest, and stomach muscles relaxed
  b Each vertebra stacked evenly one on another
  c The spine moving as a complete unit.

- Keep your shoulders, chest, and stomach muscles relaxed yet hold tension in spine.

It is of particular importance to the notion of the Celestial Stem that the spine moves as a complete unit. The Ancient masters used to say:

- The waist is the Great Commander
- Nose, navel, shoulders, and hips stay in alignment
- The body moves as a single unit
- The body leads, the arms follow.

Tips:

- Glasses affect posture by altering the position of head, so if possible leave your glasses off.
- Keep your shoulders soft – if there's tension, tap lightly between the collar bone to release.
- Think of your 'head going up and your tail going down'.

Drop The Blinds/Open The Curtains

Drop The Blinds:

- Drop your tail bone towards the ground from the point where your spine joins your hips

Open The Curtains:

- Release tension in buttocks – do not clench them!
- Important: smooth out your lower back to straighten lower spine and prevent curving like a 'duck's tail.

Carriage Movements

Opening Your Carriage

- Instead of leaning forward, shrink your 'carriage' by moving your hips backwards as though *sitting back on a chair in the dark*.

a Adopt a *Standing Like a Tree* position
b Release your knees
c Allow your hips to move slowly backwards
d Imagine *sitting back on a chair in the dark.*

Closing Your Carriage

- Reverse the motion.
- Buttocks move *as if being scooped up with a spoon* – hips, belly button leading the movement.

Protecting Your Knees, Strengthening Your Bones

Sinews-Changing Exercises

Western and Chinese (and most other Eastern) approaches to exercising the body are different in several ways. First, much of what is done in Western exercise is to strengthen the outer muscle layers. However, this is often done without strengthening the inner layers or with any attention to the connective tissue that attaches muscle to bone.

One of the most profound differences in Qigong approaches to exercising the body is the emphasis on strengthening what we in the West would call tendon, ligament and bone – which in Qigong practice are referred to as *the sinews.* The belief is that in strengthening and developing muscle without attending to making the sinews strong and supple is counterproductive and may even be harmful.

The sinews-changing exercises are a series of exercises designed to gently work and strengthen your 'sinews'. In these exercises, even more than most, positioning, placement, and architecture are of great importance.

Deviation from the directions can in fact transform the exercises from having a positive effect to a negative one. So, do please pay attention to the direction for placement, especially of your knees.

Circling Your Knees

- Begin in *Standing Post.*
- Release knees and shrink carriage – keeping your back straight and your knees touching.
- Place your hands loosely on your knees.
- Move your knees in a circle, first in one direction and then the other.

Tips:

- The movement of the knees should not go over the ends of your toes or the edges of your feet.
- Breathe naturally.

- Circle up to 32 times in each direction – if necessary, build up to this number in multiples of eight.

Precautions:

- Keep your toes and knees touching! If this is difficult, open your heels so your feet make a V shape.

Picking Up Your Toes

- Begin in *Standing Post.*
- Keep your spine straight but not rigid (see description of Celestial Stem).
- *Inhale –*
- Move your hands away from the floor

  a Thumb and fingers touching as if picking up a piece of paper
  b As you do this your elbows move away from your body.

- Simultaneously, pick your toes up towards the sky.
- *Exhale –*
- Move your hands towards the floor.
- Simultaneously, move your toes back towards the floor.

Tips:

- Do not tighten abdominal muscles.
- Keep spine relaxed.
- Imagine your hands are pulling on a string attached to your big toe.
- On exhale, release energy.

Raising Your Heels

- Begin in *Standing Post.*
- Keep your spine straight but not rigid (see description of *Celestial Stem*).
- *Inhale –*

  a Move your elbows up and away from the body, with thumbs facing your thighs
  b Simultaneously, lift your heels off the floor.

Tips:

- Move as if there is a string attached from your toes to your hands
- Do not protrude your buttocks, keep body straight.

Benefits:

- Strengthens tendons and 'exercises' the liver meridian.
- Massages heels, helps bone structure.
- Helps those with arthritis or weak joints by building strength.

Panning For Piranhas

- Begin in *Standing Post*.
- Inhale –

  a Place left palm on right shoulder just below the collar bone.

- Exhale –

  a *Shrink your carriage*

- Inhale –

  a Turn to your *right*, keeping nose and navel in alignment, and shoulders and hips in alignment.

- Exhale –

  a Return to centre.

- Repeat exercise eight times.
- Inhale –

  a Place right palm on left shoulder.

- Exhale –

  a *Shrink your carriage*

- Inhale –

  a Turn to your *left*, keeping nose and navel in alignment, and shoulders and hips in alignment.

- Exhale –

  a Return to centre.

- Repeat exercise eight times.

Precautions:

- Do not let knees extend beyond your toes
- When turning to either side, do not force the movement
- Only move as far as you can without clenching your stomach muscles

Tips:

- Move body as a single unit.
- Don't hold your breath or tighten abdominals.

Drilling For Oil

One of the quintessential Tai Chi exercises.

- Begin in *Standing Like A Tree* position.
- Slide your *right foot* forward in a straight line, stopping when your right heel is just in front of the toes of your left foot.
- Pivot on the ball of your *left foot*.
  - Move your left heel towards your right foot
  - Stop when the toes are at about a 45-degree angle.
- Move your hips backwards and relax your knees (this position is often called *Bow Stance* in Tai Chi).
- Place your palms on your hips – right palm on right hip, left palm on left hip.
- Breathe slowly and smoothly.
- Slowly and smoothly circle both knees away from the centre of your body.

VARIATION – RUNNING IN PLACE:

- Begin in *Bow Stance.*
- Alternately raise your right heel and then your left heel.
  - a Breath in while raising each heel
  - b Breath out while lowering each heel.
- Continue until tired.

Chapter 14

Adapted Exercises

Bed-Based Movement: What To Do To Improve Health When Confined To Bed

Lighting The Candle Qigong

Qigong helps lower stress levels and helps us to relax. Here is a simple Qigong exercise that can help you rest and sleep. If you wish, play soft calming music during the exercise.

- Lie back in a 'recliner' chair, or lie flat in bed.
  - a If lying in bed, place a small pillow under your head.
  - b Do not cross your legs, as this blocks circulation.
- Place your left hand, palm down, on the top of your breastbone just below your collar bone and your right hand, palm down, just below your navel.
- Allow your elbows to rest close to your body.
- Close your eyes.
- Breathe slowly and regularly through your nose – *never force or hold your breath.*
- Imagine there is a lighted candle in the space under your right hand.
- As you breathe in, imagine the flame of this candle extending upwards towards your left hand
- As you breathe out, imagine this flame returning to its original position.

Floor-Based Yoga Exercises[1]

Here are some simple examples of floor-based exercises I (BW) do regularly. They are variations on/modified versions of the 'standard'.

DOI: 10.4324/9780429439803-20

Corpse Pose (Savasana)

- Lie on your back, with your arms about 45 degrees from the sides of your body.

  a Make sure you are warm and comfortable – if you need to, place a blanket under or over your body.
  b Place a thin pillow under the back of your head.

- Close your eyes and take slow deep breaths through your nose.
- Scan your body from your toes to your fingers to your crown of your head, looking for tension, tightness, and contracted muscles. Consciously release and relax any areas that you find. If you need to, rock or wiggle parts of your body from side to side to encourage further release.
- Release all control of your breath, your mind, and your body.
- Let your body move deeper and deeper into a state of total relaxation.
- Stay in the position for a minimum of eight long slow deep breaths and for up to 15 minutes.
- When you are ready, slowly inhale up to a seated position.

Lying Butterfly Pose/Reclining Bound Angle Pose (Supta Baddha Konasana)

- Start in *Corpse Pose.*
- Breathe in slowly

  a Slowly bring your heels towards your hips with the soles of your feet touching
  b Stop when your heels are as close to your hips as is comfortable for you.

- Breathe out slowly

  a Let your knees open as wide apart as is comfortable.

- Breathe in and out naturally and slowly for eight breaths.

Balancing Table Pose (Dandayamna Bharmanasana)

- Start on your hands and knees with your back 'flat' (*Bharmanasana Table Pose*).
- Breathe in slowly

  a Slowly lifting and extending your *righ*t *leg* until it is parallel to the floor, fully stretch and point your toes away from your hips.
  b At the same time, slowly lifting and extending your *left arm* until it is parallel to the floor, fully stretch and point your fingers away from your shoulders.

- Breathe out slowly.

  a Return your leg and arm to the original *Table Pose.*

- Alternate raising right leg/left arm with left leg/right arm.
- Repeat four to ten times on each side.
- Variation: breathe in and out 2–4 times while your arm and leg are extended.

Benefits: improves balance, memory, focus and coordination. This posture builds core body strength and lengthens your spine.

Contraindications: recent or chronic injury to your knees, back, arms, or shoulders.

Floor Sun Salutation Child Pose (Balasana)

- From *Table Pose*, exhale, and lower your hips to your heels and forehead to the floor. Keep your knees together or, if more comfortable, spread the knees slightly apart.
- Your arms can be overhead with your palms on the floor, your palms or fists can be stacked under your forehead, or your arms can be alongside your body with your palms up.
- Breathe slowly and deeply, actively pressing your belly against your thighs on the inhale.
- Breathe and hold for 4–12 breaths.
- To release: place your palms under your shoulders and slowly inhale up to a seated position.

Benefits: calms your body, mind, and spirit and stimulates your third eye point. It gently stretches your low back, massages, and tones your abdominal organs, and stimulates digestion and elimination.

Contraindications: recent or chronic injury to your knees.

Modifications:

- Place a blanket under your hips, knees, and/or head.
- If you are pregnant, spread your knees wide apart to remove any pressure on your abdomen

Getting Up From Lying On Your Back On The Floor[2]

When getting up from lying down on the floor on your back, it is very important not to sit straight up quickly as this can cause a vasovagal reaction and light-headedness.

- Bring your left knee up towards your right hip.

  a Simultaneously, place your left palm up by your right shoulder.

- Turn onto your stomach and place both palms face down on the floor near your shoulders.
- Move your hips back towards your heels.
- Slide one foot forward so that your knee is parallel to the floor.
- Stand up.

Throughout this movement breathe naturally, fully, and slowly – *do not force or hold your breath.*

Wall-Based Exercises

Legs Up The Wall Pose (Viparita Karani)

- Lie flat on your back on a mat or blanket near a wall or solid door.
- Shimmy your hips as close to the wall as possible and start walking your feet up the wall.
  a Place the back of your legs against the wall, so that the soles of your feet face upwards.
  b It will take you a little bit of movement to get comfortable in this position.
- Make sure your back and head are resting on the floor so that your body forms a 90-degree angle.
  a If necessary, to make this comfortable you can
    - Place a thin pillow under your head, or
    - Let your arms rest on your belly or out to the sides.
- Close your eyes and breathe.
- Hold this position for *at least eight* full slow breaths.
- When ready, bring your knees towards your chest slowly and roll to one side.
- Breathe before you sit up.

Benefits:

- Alleviates headaches.
- Boosts energy.
- Soothes menstrual cramps, though some Yoga traditions advise against doing this during menstruation.
- Relieves lower-back pain.

Precautions:

- Glaucoma
- Hypertension
- Hernia.

Happy Baby Wall Pose (Variation On Ananda Balasana)

- Lay flat on your back on a mat or blanket near a wall or solid door.
- Place your hips as close to the wall as possible
- Place the soles of your feet on the wall about hip-width apart.
- Have your feet comfortably apart, which for you may be approximately hip-width apart.
- Allow your sacrum to sink so that it is flat on the floor.
- Let your arms rest on your belly or out to the sides.
- Close your eyes and breathe.
- Hold this position for *at least eight* full slow breaths.
- When ready, bring your knees towards your chest slowly and roll to one side.
- Breathe before you sit up.

Benefits:

- Compresses the stomach by massaging the organs in the digestive system.
- Helps reduce the heart rate by relaxing and calming the mind.

Precautions:

- To avoid injury, ensure your spine is straight.
- If you have knee injuries, be especially careful to keep them in alignment with your first toe.
- Do not practise during the late stages of pregnancy.
- People suffering from high blood pressure should not do this exercise.

Butterfly Dries Its Wings (Variation On Titli Asana)

- Lie flat on your back on a mat or blanket near a wall or solid door.

  a Your hips should be no further away from the wall than the length of your lower leg[3]

  b Your feet should be together, and the soles of your feet flat on the wall/door.

- Imagine your legs are like the winds of a butterfly resting on a wall.

The following movements are like a butterfly opening and closing its wings to dry them.

- Breathe in slowly and evenly.
- Without using force, allow your knees to open outwards with your breath.
- When you can go no further without forcing or strain, breathe out slowly and evenly.
- Moving with your breath and without using force, allow your knees to return to their original position.
- Repeat eight times.

Benefits:

- Provides a good stretch to the groin, inner thighs, and knees.
- Enhances bowel and intestine movements.
- Useful for pregnant women for a natural and healthy delivery of the child.
- Helps regulate irregular menstruation and with getting relief from menstrual discomfort.
- Beneficial for people who spend long hours walking and standing by providing relief in lower limbs.

Precautions:

- Do not force your movements!
- If you feel any strain or pain in your knee, *slowly* stretch your big toes upwards during the motion.

Counter Exercises

I regularly do the following exercises at my kitchen counter and/or my bathroom sink. The first two are variations/modifications of Yoga asanas. The second is a combination of ballet barre exercises, Kung Fu/Qigong (Flying Crane) and Yoga (Virahandrasana III/Warrior Pose III).

Half Plank Pose (Phalakasana)

This is not a true Plank Pose, hence the 'Half' in the title.

- Stand approximately 3.5–4-foot lengths from your kitchen counter.[4]
- Your feet should be

  a One-foot width apart
  b Outside edges parallel to one another.

- Breathe *in* and raise your hands above your head.
- Breath *out* and bend from the waist until your palms are flat on the kitchen counter.

- Your back should now be at 90 degrees to your hips and parallel to the floor.

  a Keep your spine straight
  b Do not raise or lower your chin as this puts a strain on your neck
  c Keep your arms shoulder-width apart with your palms flat on the counter.

- Breathe in and out normally eight times.

Cobra Pose (Bhujangasana)

- Stand in *Half Plank Pose* 3.5–4-foot lengths from your kitchen counter.

  a Keep your arms shoulder-width apart with your palms flat apart on the counter
  b Relax your elbows.

- Breathe *in*

  a Release your knees
  b Arch your spine and head fully – but do not strain or force this movement.
  c Relax your hips, belly, and chest so that they move passively towards the floor.

- Breathe *out.*
- Relax, and breathe in and out eight times.

Ballet Meets Martial Arts

- Stand in *Half Plank Pose* 3.5–4-foot lengths from your kitchen counter.
- Bring your feet together

  a Keep your arms shoulder-width apart with your palms flat on the counter.

- Breathe *in* (1)

  a Raise your right knee until your leg is parallel to the floor

    - Your toes point towards the floor.

- Breathe *out* (2)

  a Extend your leg backwards until you reach full extension

   b This creates a straight line from the tips of your toes to the tips of your fingers.

- Breathe *in* (3)

   a Bring your knee towards your chest until your leg is parallel to the floor

      - Your toes point towards the floor.

- Breathe *out* (4)

   a Drive your heel towards the floor at a 45-degree angle until your leg is straight
   b Do not lock your knee.

- Breathe *in* (5)

   a Draw your knee back towards your body until you are once again in position (1) above

- Breathe *out* (6)

   a Place your foot back on the floor until you are back at starting position.

- Repeat this sequence eight times, alternating right and left legs, i.e., four times on each side.

The quality of your breathing used in this exercise changes its intent:

- Short in-breaths with a pronounced exhale 'ha' = practice of martial arts kicks.
- Long slow breaths to the full extent of the movement = practice for dance/ballet barre.
- Holding each position for a long slow in and out breath = Qigong/Yoga practice.

Seated Exercises[5]

Tranquil Sitting

Seated exercises can be done anywhere – at home, at the office, or when travelling on a bus, in a car, or on an airplane.

Any chair will do. However, for best results choose a straight-backed armless chair.

- Sit comfortably on a chair with your legs hip width apart and your feet flat on the floor in parallel.

- Imagine there is a small cushion of air between each vertebra and that your head is suspended by a silken thread. Your chin rests on a silken pillow with your eyes parallel to the floor.
- Keep your spine straight but not rigid with your shoulders slightly forward of your hips. Do *not* tighten your stomach muscles – rather, keep the front of your body soft.

While seated, there are three essential positions for the hands:

- *Tranquil Sitting* – both palms down resting lightly on the top of the thighs.
- *Seated Wu Chi* – one hand on top of the other resting just below the navel, palms toward the body.[6]
- *Fingers Dripping Water* – arms by your side, fingers pointing towards the ground with palms facing one another.

Usually, one progresses from *Tranquil Sitting* to *Seated Wu Chi* to *Fingers Dripping Water* and finishes with *Seated Wu Chi* again. However, initially choose whichever one of the three positions feels comfortable.

- Close your mouth.
- With your teeth touching and your tongue lightly in contact with the roof of your mouth, breathe in and out through your nose, quietly and softly so that you can barely hear your breath.
- Initially maintain each position for 30 seconds to two minutes.
- Throughout your experience try to quiet your ever-questioning mind – simply sit, breathe softly, and smile.

  a Never hold or force your breath!

Grand Canyon Exercises – Seated

- Sit in *Fingers Dripping Water* position, turn your palms to face behind you.
- Inhale

  a Float your hands up in front of body until your hands are level with the top of your shoulders.

- Exhale

  a Face your palms out, your thumbs pointing to centre, fingers facing up (*Picture Frame* position).

    - Imagine you are looking at beautiful scenery – e.g., the Grand Canyon, a pristine sandy beach, a forest.

- Keep your arms straight, relax your shoulders and keep your body still.
  a Inhale and exhale three times.
- Inhale
  a Imagine a large balloon inflating – open your arms slowly and smoothly outwards about 30 degrees on each side.
- Exhale
  a Imagine the balloon deflating as you bring your arms back to the centre.
- Repeat three times.
  a Return to *Picture Frame* position.
- Inhale
  a Float your hands up about 4–6 inches.
- Exhale
- Return to *Picture Frame* position.
  a Repeat three times.
- After the third exhale return to *Seated Wu Chi.*
- *Breathe and smile* for a few moments.

Exercises While Driving The Car

Driving The Car Qigong

Qigong can be done anywhere and needs no expensive equipment. It is possible to reduce and manage your stress while driving using the following simple exercises. Doing these exercises for as little as twenty seconds at a time will help to reduce the build-up of stress and to remain alert while driving.

- Sit comfortably with your legs hip-width apart.
- When driving with cruise control, place your feet flat on the floor in parallel or rest your feet comfortably on the pedals.
- Imagine there is a 'cushion 'of air between each vertebra, that your head is suspended by a silken thread with your eyes parallel to the road.
- Keep your spine straight but not rigid.
- Relax your stomach muscles.
- Breathe in and out through your nose, quietly and softly – *never hold or force your breath!*
- Always remain alert to traffic around you.

The following positions are very helpful in reducing tension and staying alert. They also aid in developing your peripheral vision.

The hand positions described refer to the analog 12-hour clock. For both positions, imagine holding a driving wheel softly (do not grip tightly) and breathe smoothly and naturally.

Universal Post

- Place your hands at ten and two on the clock (ten minutes to two position).
- Relax your shoulders.
- Imagine there is a small orange under your armpits so that your arms are slightly away from your chest.
- Your elbows point towards the ground.

This position helps to slow pulse rate and regulate blood pressure. It is particularly beneficial whenever your car is stationary (e.g., in a traffic jam or at the lights).

Lotus Blossom Floating On Water

- Place your hands at seven and five on the clock (25 minutes past seven position).
- Palms facing upwards and towards your navel.
- Relax your shoulders.
- Your elbows point away from your body.

This position helps to draw in energy and calm the mind. It is particularly suitable when driving long distances.

As the saying goes, 'a heart attack is only one heartbeat away'. So, when driving, simply breathe softly and smile.

Notes

1 For more information on 'starter' Yoga exercises I recommend the following: Yoga Basics, www.yogabasics.com/; S. Powers (2008), *Insight Yoga: An Innovative Synthesis of Traditional Yoga, Meditation, and Eastern Approaches to Healing and Well-Being* (Boulder, CA: Shambhala).
2 This an adaptation of a Laban exercise.
3 Lower leg = tibia/fibula.
4 This can also be done outside on the balcony of a ship or a flat/apartment using the rail instead of the kitchen counter.
5 The exercises that follow are included in my *Breathe and Smile Seated Qigong* video: www.youtube.com/watch?v=poFZmMSbqGA
6 Traditional Chinese medicine states that men should place their left hand closest to the body and women their right.

Chapter 15

Walking For Health

The Health Benefits Of Walking

Over the last fifty years, modern life has become faster. Life and job stresses have increased. People now eat larger portions, walk less, and there is an alarming rise in obesity and stress-related diseases. We rely more on cars and sit in front of our computers and TVs a great deal more. Our sedentary life is literally slowly killing us.

Walking is one of the best forms of exercise. When you walk you carry your own body weight, and the heavier you are the more calories you burn when walking the same distance. It may seem too good to be true, but making the decision to get off the couch and go for a walk is the first step towards a healthy and potentially longer life.

Walking is becoming an increasingly popular intervention for getting fitter and losing weight, as well as helping with stress. Walking 10,000 steps, which equates to about two hours of walking, will result in the burning of approximately 400 calories or up to 2,800 calories per week. Regular walking can help lower the rate of weight gain; strengthen memory; and protect you from heart disease.

Research suggests some of the benefits of walking include[1,2,3,4]:

- Increased cardiovascular and pulmonary (heart and lung) fitness
- Reduced risk of heart disease and stroke
- Improved management of conditions such as hypertension (high blood pressure), high cholesterol, joint and muscular pain or stiffness, and diabetes
- Stronger bones and improved balance
- Increased muscle strength and endurance
- Reduced body fat
- Significantly reduce mortality in older adults.

Conventional Western wisdom suggests that to gain the maximum health benefits you should walk for at least thirty minutes briskly, meaning that you can still talk but not sing, at least three times a week. While this may be true,

DOI: 10.4324/9780429439803-21

the benefits of walking can accrue from simply getting 'off the couch' and going for slower and more leisurely strolls.

In addition to the obvious walking practice of simply putting one foot in front of the other, there are many other different styles of walking.[5,6] Chinese martial arts practice employs multiple ways of stepping and walking. Underlying these movements is Qigong. While 'Qigong' is a modern construct, many of the methods that are used today are derived from age-old Chinese traditions – most notably Taoist and Buddhist longevity (so called immortality) techniques, meditations, and martial arts training exercises.

As mentioned elsewhere in this book, these exercises emphasise the cultivation of internal energy by focusing on breathing patterns, physical posture, and coordination that help stimulate hormone secretion, immune function, and oxygenation of body cells. All of which help to promote health and counter stress and stress-related illnesses.

A Journey Of A Thousand Miles Begins With A Single Step

There are many techniques which help magnify the beneficial effects of simple walking. These include swinging your arms and linking your breath to the walk ––and very specific arm postures that influence different bodily processes and organs.

Basic walking is a great start. Integrating Qigong-based walking patterns takes this further as these help prevent illness, improve the supply of nutrients and oxygen in your body, and remove toxins and waste material efficiently.

The mindful practice of Qigong-based walking takes your focus off conscious distractions and the stressors of everyday life, helping to alleviate *situational stress.*

The rhythmic movements and breathing allow your body, without conscious thought, to start to reduce *insipient stress*, those everyday micro stresses which like extra layers of clothing have been weighing you down throughout your life.

Qigong Walks

The following exercises are excellent for improving balance, poise, and coordination.

Shifting Weight

Throughout this exercise:

- Keep your spine straight and your head erect:

  a Do not collapse (fold) at the centre
  b Do not bob your head up and down.

- *Exhale* as you move to the side.
- *Inhale* as you move towards centre.

To begin:

- Stand in the *Standing Like A Tree* position.
- Inhale.
- As you exhale, slowly shift your weight onto your left side so that 80% of your weight is over your left leg with your knee slightly bent and directly over your foot.

  a Hold this position for a second or two.

- Slowly transfer your weight first to the centre and then to your right side so that 80% of your weight is over your right leg with your knee slightly bent and directly over your foot.

  a Hold this position for a second or two.

- Return to centre.

Walking On Thin Ice: Polishing The Floor (Basic Qigong Walk)

Throughout this exercise:

- Keep your spine straight and your head erect throughout this exercise

  a Do not collapse (fold) at the centre
  b Do not bob your head up and down.

- *Exhale* as you move to the side.
- *Inhale* as you move towards centre.

To begin:

- Stand in the *Standing Like A Tree* position.
- Shift all your weight onto your left side

  a Imagine you have a soft cloth under your right foot
  b Keep the sole of your right foot parallel to the floor.

- Circle your foot first clockwise and then anticlockwise

  a Moving the soft cloth as you do so and varying the size of the circles you make.

- Then shift all your weight onto your right side and make circles with your left foot.

Walking On Thin Ice II: Walking In The Dark (Basic Qigong Walk)

In this exercise your feet move in alternate semicircles with your weight shifting first from one side of your body to the other. Throughout the exercise:

- Try not to bob your head up and down as you walk.
- *Inhale* as you shift your weight onto one side.
- *Exhale* as you arc your foot across the floor.

To begin:

- Stand in the *Standing Like A Tree* position.
- Shift all your weight onto your left side.
- Move your right foot out and forward clockwise in a semi-circular arc
    a Your foot should remain parallel to the floor as in *Polishing The Floor* above.
- When your right foot has travelled 180 degrees and reached a point straight in front of its original position, shift all your weight onto your right side.
- When your weight is fully on your right side, move your left foot out and forward in an anti-clockwise semi-circular arc.
    a Again, parallel to the floor as in *Polishing The Floor* above.
- When your left foot has travelled 180 degrees and has reached a point ahead of your right foot and straight in front of its previous position, shift your weight on to your left foot.
- Continue moving forward in this fashion.
    a Work towards making the coordination of the shifting of weight from one side to the other with the arcing movement of one foot after another as smooth and fluid as possible.

Guo Lin Qigong – Anti-Cancer Walk

One example of Qigong-based walking practices that have been documented to help alleviate stress and stress related illness, is the *Anti-Cancer Walk* developed by Madam Guo Lin.

Guo Lin was one of the most famous female Qigong masters of the 20th century. However, in 1949 she was diagnosed with cervical cancer. She underwent Western medical treatment. She had a hysterectomy, chemotherapy, and radiation. She developed further metastatic disease and experienced a total of seven operations within ten years. However, after suffering another major relapse and being told she had only six months to live, she revisited the Qigong her grandfather had taught her as a child. Her subsequent research into ancient writings on Qigong practices helped her develop her own walking regime. This regime came to be known as *Guo Lin Qigong*, or, more colloquially, the *Madam Guo Lin Anti-Cancer Walk.* Within six months of practising this for two hours each day, her cancer went into remission.[7]

This walk has three parts:

- *Breathing Like the Wind*
- *Bear Shuffling Through the Woods*
- *Raising the Wet Cloth.*

The great effects of this exercise are achieved through coordination and synchronisation of your movements with your breathing as you walk slowly forward raising your arms to the same side as you twist your body.

This walk is perhaps easier to learn if you practise each of its three parts separately.

(1) *Breathing Like the Wind* – breathing technique:

- Breathe through your nose in the following pattern:

  a Short in-breath,
  b Short in-breath,
  c Long out-breath.

(2) *Bear Shuffles Through the Woods* – walking technique:

- Move slowly forward in the following manner:

  a Lift your right heel – coordinate with a short in-breath.
  b Lift right foot – coordinate with a short in-breath.
  c Place right foot on floor – heel through toe – coordinate with a long out-breath.
  d Repeat pattern on the left side.
  e NB: heel of moving foot is placed at same level as the big toe of planted foot.

(3) *Raising the Wet Cloth* – twisting the body technique:

- Part A
- Imagine you are picking up a piece of wet silk cloth or pre-pasted wallpaper.

  a Relax stomach, back straight, using legs for balance
  b First three fingers almost touch as you lift hands up in front of body to eyebrow height

c Keep wrists curved but relaxed as they rise to eyebrow level.

- At eyebrow level, raise your fingers so that your palms are flat and facing away from you.
- Slowly move your arms down towards the floor as though you are mopping wallpaper to a wet glass screen.
- When your hands reach navel level, repeat sequence from picking up wet cloth.

a Make sure you exhale as you 'mop down'.

- Part B
- Follow directions for part A, but

a As you raise your arms, slowly use your waist to turn your shoulders and hips away from your centre to the *right*, keeping your arms in front of your body.
b As you lower your arms, turn your body slowly from the waist back to centre.
c Repeat on the *left* side.

Throughout the exercise:

- Your hips initiate the movement, allowing your arms to swing from side to side.
- Your hands do not go above hip level.
- Your knees do not bounce.

This style of walking is best practised in the morning outside near water or under trees. But, as with any Qigong exercise, the benefits can be experienced anywhere and at any time of the day.

This practice is best done for up to two hours a day as 15-minute sessions of walking with breaks in between. However, you can start by taking a few steps, then stopping and resting, then another few steps, and so on. Gradually, as stamina improves you can build up the length of time you are able to walk.

A great deal has been written about the effectiveness of *Guo Lin Qigong* and overall, it does appear to be an effective complementary therapeutic approach. Studies have shown it to improve quality of life and decrease depression and anxiety – all of which are important to the mind-body connection which strongly influences how a cancer patient responds to treatment.[8]

Benefits Of Walking In A Circle[9,10,11]

Another example of a health-promoting Qigong walk is drawn from Bagua Zhang. *Circle Walking* is the quintessential exercise. When I (BW) first encountered this practice I asked my teacher, Master Hu, how long I should perform it. He suggested that I start with *1,000 circles in each direction.* I thought he was joking – he wasn't! He placed a large plastic garbage bin in the centre of the gym and instructed me to walk in a circle around it. I still have the video!

Circle Walking is a powerful non-aerobic cardiovascular exercise that can be practised regularly anywhere. It can range from being at home, in a relatively small space, by pushing back furniture, to any open space outdoors. It does not matter what you use as the focal point of your circle.

Ba Gua Circle Walking helps:

- Engage and massage your internal organs – especially the kidneys and bowels
- Improve the functioning of your vascular system.
- Strengthen your muscles
- Improve balance
- Reduce stress
- Boost the immune system
- Eliminate toxins
- Increase flexibility
- Improve cardiovascular health.

All of which are incredibly important not simply for combatting stress but also in improving overall health and vitality.

Opening – Fierce Tiger Escapes From Cave

- Stand with your feet together

  a Hips relaxed backward
  b Knees released.

- Palms face down, fingers slightly apart.
- Hands are at hip level.
- 'Balls' of energy under armpits.
- Elbows slightly bent facing out to the sides.

Circle Walking

- Begin by moving *counter-clockwise* (turn to your *left*).
- Start with your feet together.
- Turn your hips slightly towards the centre of the circle.
- Move your *right* (outside) foot forward in a circular motion.
- Then drive your *left* (inside) foot forward in a straight line

  a Until it is parallel with the right foot.

- Turn at the waist slightly as you walk

  a *Do not place weight on pivoting leg!*

- To avoid strain on your knees, transfer weight to your turning leg as you move.

Sixteen steps usually complete a full circle.

- To change direction and move *clockwise* (turn to your *right*).
- Come to a complete stop with your feet together.
- Turn your hips slightly towards the centre of the circle
- Move your *left* foot forward in a circular motion towards the centre of the circle.
- Then drive your *right* foot forward in a straight line.
- Then move as above.

Carry the Baby (Left)

- As for *moving counter-clockwise* above.
- As you turn your hips towards the centre of the circle

  a Move your hands across your body at hip height until your *left* hand is in the centre of the circle and your *right* hand rests at your *left* hip.

- Turn both palms up

  a Imagine you are supporting a baby's head in your right palm and its bottom in your left palm.

- Continue *Circle Walking* as described above.

Lion Opens Its Mouth

- Palms turn in toward each other, as if a ball is between them, fingers facing wrist of opposite hand, right hand on top.
- As you turn, the arms (the lion's mouth) opens, until they are wide enough to hold a large medicine ball to one side.
- Elbows slightly point down as arms and hands open so right arm is above head and left hand is down around hip area.
- Left thumb and right little finger are connected (start with touching, move further apart, drop right elbow/opening from left elbow).
- You may feel as though you are leaning slightly forward, if so, be sure to turn eyes up.

Notes

1 Ideas in this chapter were first explored in B. Warren and C. Hind (2020), A Journey of a Thousand Steps: Qigong Walks for Health. *International Journal of Complementary and Alternative Medicine* 13(1): 31–34. www.researchgate.net/publication/339828548_A_Journey_of_A_Thousand_Steps_Qigong_Walks_for_Health
2 K. Asp (2022), www.realsimple.com/health/fitness-exercise/benefits-walking#walking-9
3 A. Glasper (2017), https://pubmed.ncbi.nlm.nih.gov/28345987/
4 Better Health Victoria (nd), www.betterhealth.vic.gov.au/health/healthyliving/walking-for-good-health
5 Sheng Ken Yun (1997), *Walking Kung* (Red Wheel/Weiser).
6 J. MoraMarco and R. Benzel (2000), *The Way of Walking* (Chicago: Contemporary Books).
7 Qigong Chinese Health (nd), www.qigongchinesehealth.com/walking_qigong
8 W. Wang et al. (1996), https://books.google.ca/books?hl=en&lr=&id=1YnP0Jx-QvIC&oi=fnd&pg=PA209&dq=Walking+Qigong+Guo+Lin&ots=tAjvukXWZV&sig=j2HFyYquEOcxVG4EBYAauyzhhTY#v=onepage&q&f=false
9 S. Painter (nd), https://feng-shui.lovetoknow.com/Bagua_Circle
10 B. Frantzis (2010), www.energyarts.com/bagua-circle-walking/
11 T. Bisio (2012), www.internalartsinternational.com/free/the-perfect-exercise-ba-gua-circle-walking-nei-gong/

Chapter 16

Breathe, Smile, Stretch

Brief Eastern Routines For Busy People

Modern life and efforts to achieve work-life balance can often make it difficult to find enough time to exercise. The good news is that recent research suggests that short bursts of activity done several times during a day are just as, if not more, beneficial that one long session.[1,2,3,4] For example, several short walks throughout a day are at least as effective as one continuous bout of the same total duration in reducing cardiovascular risk and improving aspects of mood in previously sedentary individuals.[5]

I (BW) started to go favour short bursts of exercise just after my daughter was born. I realised I could not in good conscience take an hour or more to do my regular morning martial arts practice. So, I would find a quiet space for a 1–5-minute break from parenting. Outside when it was warm enough, but anywhere would do when too cold, and always aided and abetted by my cat Grand Master Tikka.[6]

I have now retired, and I do not want the lack of exercise to reduce my mobility and affect my health. However, this does not mean I don't still exercise in short bursts when I do not have enough time for a full workout session. Here are a few of my brief workout activities.

One-Minute Exercises

White Crane Stretches To The Heavens

The white crane is revered in many cultures throughout the world as a symbol of stability, wisdom, and fidelity. In Chinese mythology, cranes are generally symbolically connected with the idea of immortality and Taoist 'immortals' were said to have magical abilities to transform into cranes to fly on various journeys.

This exercise provides a full body stretch and energises the body. It can be done anywhere, but a tranquil spot facing water enhances its benefits.

- Begin in *Standing Post* stance, with

DOI: 10.4324/9780429439803-22

a Feet together
b Arms by your side – palms towards your thighs.

- *Slowly inhale*

  a As you inhale, slowly stand up while moving your arms slowly outwards away from your body upwards towards the sky.

  - Continue until the backs of your hands meet above your head.
  - As your arms move upwards, slowly tilt your head upwards as you breathe.

- When your arms are extended as far as you can go and your head is tilted upwards, hold pose before continuing breathing.
- *Slowly exhale*

  a As you exhale, bend your knees and slowly shrink your carriage, folding your body as you move towards the floor.

  - Let your head return to its normal resting point
  - Your arms circle downwards towards the floor.

- Repeat eight times.

Placing The Needle At The Bottom Of The Sea

- Begin in the *Inverted Y* posture.
- Inhale
- Exhale

  a Move your hips backwards allowing your chest to move downwards
  b Simultaneously, place the backs of your hands together in front of your body and continue the motion towards the floor as far as possible without bending your knees.

- Inhale

  a Keeping your back straight, gently rock your hips forward, returning you to *Inverted Y.*
  b Continue the motion until your chest faces the sky.
  c Simultaneously, your hands open from the Dan Tien, extending to the side of your body with your palms facing towards the sky.
  d Fold your arms in towards the Dan Tien.

- Exhale

  a Flip your palms over

- Return to beginning and repeat 3–5 times.

Tips:

- Do not lean forward at the chest; keep your spine straight
- Only go as far as you are able without straining or hurting
- Do not bounce
- Breathe smoothly and slowly
- Move smoothly and slowly

Precautions:

- Do not over-extend your range of motion.
- Do not lock any joints – *locking blocks energy.*

2–3-Minute Exercises

Grand Canyon Exercise

(1) *Picture Frame*

- Stand in *Inverted Y* position.
- Inhale
    - a Float your hands up in front of body until your hands are level with the top of your shoulders.
- Exhale
    - a Turn your wrists so that the palms face away from your body, your thumbs pointing to centre, fingers facing up (*Picture Frame* position).
    - b Imagine you are looking at beautiful scenery – e.g., the Grand Canyon, a pristine sandy beach, a forest.
- Keep your arms straight, relax your shoulders, and keep your body still.
    - a Inhale and exhale three times.
- Inhale
    - a Imagine a large balloon inflating – open your arms slowly and smoothly outwards about 30 degrees on each side.
- Exhale
    - a Imagine the balloon deflating as you bring your arms back to the centre.
- Repeat three times.
- Return to *Picture Frame* position.
- Inhale

a Float your hands up about 4–6 inches.

- Exhale

  a Return to *Picture Frame* position.

- Repeat three times.

(2) *Buddha Holds The Walls*

- Inhale

  a Extend arms to the sides until wrists are in line with the shoulder (*Buddha Holds The Walls*).

- Exhale

  a Relax shoulders.

- Inhale

  a Move 30 degrees to middle.

- Exhale

  a Return to *Buddha Holds The Walls.*

- Repeat three times.

(3) *Buddha Climbs The Walls*

- Inhale

  a Lift arms 4–6 inches (*Buddha Climbs The Walls*) from *Buddha Holds The Walls* position.

- Exhale

  a Return to *Buddha Hold The Walls.*

- Repeat three times.

Tips:

- For *Picture Frame* and *Buddha* positions, extend arms as far as you can go without locking wrists, elbows, or shoulders – locking joints blocks energy.

(4) *Turtle Breathing*

- Inhale

  a Drop wrists so that palms face the ground.

- Exhale
  - a Hips move backwards and arms fold in towards hips until hands come to rest on your lower back at hip height (*Turtle* position).
- Inhale
  - a Simultaneously, raise your body back towards *Inverted Y* while moving your hands away from your hips
- Exhale
  - a Return to *Turtle* position.
- Repeat three times
  - a After the third repetition, return to *Inverted Y.*
- Breathe and smile for a few moments.

(5) *Lifting Weights*

- Inhale
  - a Move your elbows away from your body, raising your middle finger up the side of your body towards your armpit, rotate wrists so that your wrists face the ground and thumbs touch sides of the body.
- Exhale
  - a slowly lower hands back to Inverted Y
- Repeat three times.

(6) *Inflating A Balloon*

- Breathe naturally.
- Keeping your elbows relaxed and near your body, raise hands so that palms are facing your belly button.
- Inhale
  - a Palms move away from the body.
- Exhale
  - a Palms return to body.

Tips:

- Imagine your palms resting on the outside of a balloon.

- As you *inhale*, balloon inflates, and as you *exhale*, it returns to its original size.
- Keep shoulders and elbows relaxed.

Yi Chuan/Zhan Zhuang – Simple Energy Circle

Stand Like a Tree, Flow Like Water

Yi Chuan (or *Zhan Zhuang*), the so-called 'Iron Shirt' training exercises for building strong bones and muscles, is based on the Chinese theory: sky above, earth below, and man stands like a tree rooted between the two.

Each pose may be held for as briefly as three slow breaths. This takes approximately 2–5 minutes. However, if you have more time the sequence can be longer, with each pose held for 2–5 minutes.

(1) *Standing Like A Tree – Hands Resting On Your Belly*

- Adopt *Standing Like A Tree* position
  - a Legs hip-width apart – approximately one-foot between the arches of your two feet
  - b Feet flat on the floor, parallel to one another
  - c Knees bent, but not extended beyond your toes
  - d Shoulders relaxed and spine *straight but not rigid.*
- Your eyes look at a point in the distance that is parallel to the ground.
- Move your hips slightly backwards as if sitting down on a high bar stool or a horse so that your shoulders are slightly forward of your hips.
- Point your elbows slightly away from your body with your palms facing towards your body resting on your belly button
  - a Do not tighten your stomach muscles – rather, keep the front of your body soft.
- Continue breathing naturally for eight long slow breaths.

(2) *Resting Both Hands On A Ball In The Water*

- Inhale
  - a Imagine a small balloon inflating as you slowly move your hands away from your body.
  - b Continue until your hands are about 8–10 inches away from your body.
  - c As you do so turn your palms to face the floor – fingers almost touching.

d Imagine that your palms are resting on a soccer ball on top of a stream.

- Continue breathing naturally for eight long slow breaths.

(3) *Pushing A Soccer Ball Away From Your Chest*

- Inhale

a Slowly raise your arms upwards and away from your body.
b Stop when your hands are about heart height, your palms facing away from your body.
c Imagine that your palms are lightly pushing a soccer ball away from your chest.

- Continue breathing naturally for eight long slow breaths.

(4) *Protecting Your Face*

- Inhale

a Raise your hands upwards in a circular movement.
b Straighten your legs while simultaneously leaning backwards.
c Stop raising your hands when they reach eyebrow level.
d Imagine your hands stop a soccer ball from hitting your face.

- Continue breathing naturally for eight long slow breaths.

(5) *Carrying The World On Your Chest*

- Inhale

a Slowly open your arms until they are wide enough to contain a very large ball, your palms facing towards the sky.
b Lower until your elbows are at shoulder height.
c Imagine you are holding the world – supporting it with your chest, forehead, and palms.

- Continue breathing naturally for eight long slow breaths.

(6) *Resting Your Hands On Two Balloons In The Stream*

- Inhale

a Move your arms downwards and outwards until your palms are at hip height, slightly in front of the body and facing downwards.
b Imagine under each hand you are lightly pressing a ball on top of a stream.

- Continue breathing naturally for eight long slow breaths.

(7) Return to *Standing Like A Tree – Hands Resting On Your Belly*

- Continue breathing naturally for eight long slow breaths.

Benefits: you can practise this even if you only have thirty seconds. The pose can also be adopted while waiting for a bus or train or at an airport.

While the body does not move during the exercises at an advanced level, ancient masters used to say the mind Yi (Yee) leads Chi (Chee) through the meridians of the body, cleansing and strengthening as it goes.

Notes

1 M.H. Murphy et al. (2019), https://link.springer.com/article/10.1007/s40279-019-01145-2
2 P.H. Saint-Maurice et al. (2018), www.ahajournals.org/doi/10.1161/JAHA.117.007678
3 L. Campbell et al. (2010), www.ncbi.nlm.nih.gov/pmc/articles/PMC3737972/
4 S. Lindberg (2021), www.healthline.com/health/fitness/fit-it-in-mini-workouts#exercise-guidelines
5 M.H. Murphy et al. (2002), https://wlv.openrepository.com/handle/2436/11110
6 Grand Master Tikka's adventures can be found in my illustrated book, *Teddy Teaches Tai Chi* (2022).

Chapter 17

Cool-Down Exercises

At the end of each Eastern session, it is always a good idea to do some cool down exercises. These help regulate the flow of blood through the capillaries and energy through the meridians.

Here are a few simple cool down exercises. Each one addresses blood and energy flow through specific areas of the body. Done as a set they help blood and energy flow throughout the body, helping to keep all systems and body functions in balance.

Dry Washing Exercises

Dry Washing Your Face And Hair

- Begin in *Standing Like A Tree*
- Breathe in and clap and then rub your hands together until they feel warm.
- Place your hands on your face

    a Using the tips of your fingers, move your hands slightly downwards

    - Towards your chin, then
    - Towards the base of your earlobe, then
    - Across the forehead, past the top of your ear.

- Inhale

    a Raise your elbow, and draw your fingertips backwards across your head until you reach your shoulders.

- Exhale

    a Continue the motion down the front of the body until you reach your ankles.

- Inhale

DOI: 10.4324/9780429439803-23

a Circle around your ankles and continue the movement up the back of your legs until you reach the lower back.

- Repeat three times.

Cleaning The Coat

(a) *Cleaning The Inside Of The Coat*

- Begin in *Standing Like A Tree.*
- Hold one arm out to the side, arm raised slightly, palm pointing toward the sky

  a Relax the elbow and shoulder.

- Inhale

  a Using your fingertips of the arm *not* raised, lightly brush the extended arm from the tips of the fingers to the shoulder.

- Exhale

  a Continue the motion down the centre of the body.

- Repeat 3–5 times.

(b) *Cleaning The Outside Of The Coat*

- Inhale

  a Starting from the belly button, lightly touching with your fingertips, raise up the centre line of the body to the shoulder.

- Exhale

  a Continue the motion down the outside of your arm, past your elbow and down your little finger

- Repeat 3–5 times.
- Repeat above process on other arm.

Benefits:

- This exercise helps release tension in the wrists (helpful to release tension caused by a lot of typing)
- It also aids circulation and helps avoid bruising.

Warming Your Shoulders

- Begin in *Standing Like A Tree.*
- Breathe naturally

  a Place palm underneath the collar bone and circle your hand until the area becomes warm.

- Inhale

  a Inhale to the shoulder.

- Exhale

  a Draw hand across the collar bone to the breastbone and down the front of the body.

- Repeat exercise on opposite side.
- Repeat up to three times on each side.

Cleaning Sword Sash

- Begin in *Standing Like A Tree.*
- Inhale

  a Fold arm across body until fingers touch opposite shoulder.

- Exhale

  a Draw fingers across body in a diagonal from shoulder to opposing hip.

Self-Massage

Self-Hug

- Begin in *Standing Like A Tree.*
- Cross your arms at chest height to give yourself a hug.
- Inhale

  a Circle your head upwards and to the right.

- Exhale

  a Head continues the circle down and to the left.

- Repeat 3–5 times.
- Repeat in other direction – i.e., head circles to the left.

Owie, Owie

- Begin in *Standing Like A Tree.*
- Place the first (index) finger alongside the inner thumb next to the nail

  a This raises the knuckle.

- Place raised knuckle at the glabella (point where the base of the nose joins the upper lip).
- Draw small circles.
- Repeat until it hurts.

Benefits:

- Helps release tension at the back of the neck.
- Helps relieve sinus congestion.

Tapping Your Chest

- Begin in *Standing Like A Tree.*
- Breathe naturally

  a Touch your index and middle fingers together and place on the top of your breastbone (Breathing Point 3, Tiantu).

- Tap on the top of the breastbone.

Benefits:

- Helps release tension at the back of the neck.
- Can be used to help relieve asthma, chest congestion (bronchitis), coughs.

Like A Chicken Qi Gong

- Begin in *Standing Like A Tree.*
- Place your hands at your armpit area.
- Inhale

  a Arms circle up and to the back.

- Exhale

  a Arms drop back down to the starting position.

- Repeat 3–5 times.
- Reverse.

Tips:

- Arms should create a 'wing'.
- Circle slowly and smoothly.

Line-Backer Qi Gong

- Begin in *Standing Like A Tree.*
- Inhale smoothly
  - a Raise your shoulders up towards your ears.
- Exhale smoothly
  - a Lower shoulders down.
- Repeat three times.
- Repeat above exercise using three staccato breaths.

Tip: imagine shrugging.

Shake Hands Qi Gong

- Stand in *Standing Like A Tree.*
- Breathe naturally, keeping shoulders and elbows relaxed.
- Place hands at waist height facing one another
  - a Shake hands from the wrist in front of body
    - Both hands to one side of body
    - Move across body to other side
    - Hands separately on each side of body
    - One hand to the front and one to the back, reverse.

Tassel Dance

- Lift hands to chest height
  - a Circle wrists towards each other
  - b Circle wrists away from each other.

Playing The Piano Badly

- Turn hands so that palms are towards the floor at waist height
  - a Shake hands up and down, as if playing a piano badly.

Changing Light Bulbs

- Raise your arms until your hands are above your head with your palms facing one another and your fingers pointing to the sky.

  a Rotate your wrists as if screwing in a light bulb.

- Continue the motion while slowly lowering your arms to waist height.
- At waist height, start bringing your hands back towards your body

  a Slowly move your arms towards your sides
  b Shake your hands towards the ground.

Milk The Cow

- Starting with the little finger of your left hand, lightly grasp your little finger with your right hand.
- Using a circular motion, gently pull away from the body.

  a Repeat this motion on all fingers of the left hand.

- Continue these actions starting with the thumb of your right hand.
- These actions can be repeated as many times as you want.

Tip: imagine shaking water off of hand.
Benefits:

- Helps with blood flow to the extremities.
- Helps with the prevention and amelioration of arthritis.

Massaging Your Legs

- Begin in *Standing Like A Tree.*
- Inhale

  a Place your hands on your belly.

- Exhale

  a Slowly move your palms downwards from your belly button down the inside of your thigh to the front of your knees.

- Inhale

  a Circle your hands around your knees and up around the outside edge of your thighs
  b Bring your hands back up towards the centre.

- Exhale

  a Move your hands down the middle of your thighs.

- Inhale

  a Circle around your knees and continue up the back of your thighs
  b Bring your hands back up towards the centre.

- Inhale

  a Swing your arms upwards and cross them at chest height.

- Exhale

  a Swing arms downwards and away from the body.

- Simultaneously, on the in-breath, raise a knee and one exhale return your foot to the floor
- Alternate knees as if marching for 3–5 breaths
- Come to rest in *Standing Like a Tree*
- Open your fingers and breathe naturally for 3–5 breaths.

Energy Cleansing Exercises

Cleansing The Body

- Begin in *Standing Like a Tree.*
- Inhale

  a Fold your arms in towards your belly (Breathing Point 1).

- Exhale

  a Move your hands down the inside of your thighs, lowering all the way to your ankles
  b Circle your ankle.

- Inhale

  a Come back up the back of your legs from your heels to your lower back.

- Exhale

  a Move your hands out away from your body while brushing your lower back.

- Repeat the above motion with the centre of the chest (Breathing Point 2).
- Follow this with the top of the chest (Breathing Point 3).

Massaging Your Ribs and Kidneys

- Begin in *Standing Like a Tree.*
- Rub your palms together until they are warm.
- Place your palms on your body, directly beneath your rib cage

    a Breathe naturally and circle your hands down and out.

- Continue this circular motion as you move your hands past your sides to your lower back.
- Move your hands back towards the *Dan Tien* and rest your hands on your belly.

Benefit: this is reputed to help prevent cancer.

Sealing Energy

- Begin in *Standing Like a Tree.*
- Breathe naturally
- Fold your hands into your belly so that your palms are one on top of the other

    a Circle hands around belly in clockwise direction, gradually making circles larger
    b Reverse direction and gradually return to resting your hands on your belly.

- Take three slow, smooth breaths.
- Return to *Standing Like a Tree.*

Elephants Stomp Their Feet

- Begin in *Standing Post.*
- Breathe naturally.
- Lift one foot and then the other off the ground, as if marching on the spot.
- At the same time *swing* your arms up and down in front of your body

    a Both palms facing towards the ground
    b One hand on top of the other.

- Alternate which hand is on top with each new stomp.

Benefit: this exercise helps regulate the flow of Chi throughout all the meridians.

Part VI

Western Exercises: Moving With The Universe

In this section, the authors build on ideas introduced in part V but from a more familiar Western perspective. Each chapter describes in detail specific exercises to help reduce stress, deal with little physical ailments, and prevent injuries. The exercises are geared towards individuals, but many can also be used with groups.

DOI: 10.4324/9780429439803-24

Chapter 18

From Stasis To Movement

Preparing Your Space For Action

Elsewhere in this book we have already written about how space affects mood and social interactions and how to prepare your small spaces for Qigong and Yoga. The comments made in those sections also apply to the exercises presented in this section.

As some of the exercises described below require larger space than most Eastern exercises, pay particular attention to the following points:

- Move back all furniture to create as large an open space as possible.
- Make sure that any sharp edges and breakable objects are well away from your movement area.
    a If you have a ceiling fan, switch it off and try not raise your hand too high under it.
- Sweep, vacuum, mop the floor before you start moving.
- Wear soft shoes e.g., light dance shoes, or water shoes, or go barefoot
    a Heavy shoes even runners/trainers tend to restrict movement.
- It is important to open a window(s) to let in fresh air even on the coldest winter day.

Top Tips For Daily Movement: From Western Practice

We spend too much time in semi-stasis. Before moving from these immobile positions to standing and walking, we need a *transition* period that allows the body to 'reboot' – we need to warm up the body, do some 'serious wiggling', to prepare for the sudden change into movement.

The following are some quick tips for transitioning from relative stasis to movement: what to do, what to avoid, and why.

DOI: 10.4324/9780429439803-25

- Push from the *heels* (not further forward on the foot) when going from sitting to standing, on climbing stairs, pushing, or lifting something heavy.
- When bending or walking, be sure your knees are directly in line with and over the centre of your foot.
- When bending your knees, be sure never to extend them beyond the end of the big toes (hinge hips out backward further if needed to prevent this).
- *Breathe with the movement*:

  a Breathing with the movement, especially synchronising your breathing with your movement, greatly reduces the chances of pulling, straining, spraining, tearing, or breaking ligaments, tendons, muscles, bones, etc.

    - e.g., in ballet, a grand jeté or a lift in a pas de deux; in basketball, a jump shot.

  b Always *exhale* 'on the effort'
  c *Never* hold your breath
  d *Never* breathe against the movement
  e Breathe from your diaphragm, not just your upper lungs.

- To bend over for something, or to lower yourself onto the ground, 'hinge' or 'fold' the body rather than 'bending' over...create a 'zig-zag' with hips hinged back to counter knees and ankles bent (but knees never further forward than big toes).

In addition, employ *transitional wiggling*:

- Before lurching to standing from lying down or from chairs after long sitting, 'wiggle' everything: feet, ankles, knees, hips, shoulders, arms, torso, neck, and head.
- Move in as many ways possible: bend, twist, flex, circle ...'wiggle' the entire body *gently* but completely while still in the resting position. Only then, begin to move to standing.

These transitional 'wiggles' can be done discreetly, but effectively, even when preparing to leave a business meeting, or get up and moving in any public other gathering. Once you start to incorporate these transitional 'wiggle' moments into daily practice, you will quickly notice how much easier and more fluid your movements become.

Benefits:

- Allows tendons, muscles, and joints to 'warm up'
- Assures more even blood flow and circulation throughout the whole body, thereby lessening chances of trips, falls or stumbles.

- Avoids re-injuring or re-stressing areas of present or former injuries or weakness
- Helps alleviate arthritic joint pain, stiff joints from age, inactivity, too much travel, etc.

Resetting Occasional 'Niggles': Stepping Back To Move Forward

Occasionally, on getting up to walk, we find that we get sudden aches, 'kinks', or pain in ankles, feet, toes, or knees. The pain doesn't seem to indicate an injury or serious condition, but it's annoying and prevents us from moving in a pain-free manner.

A Suggested Response

Sometimes we can inadvertently come up with a 'fix' that works – especially if we are prepared to experiment and watch out for happy successful accidents.

- When these sudden aches appear and affect gait, simply take two or three steps straight backward, then resume your forward walk.
- You may find that, 'somehow,' the niggles have gone – at least for a while.
- If they return, simply do the backward steps again.

There may be a simple kinaesthetic rationale, which I do not have, but I know from my own and others' anecdotal experience that this 'move backward to go forward' can provide fast, simple, effective relief for those 'niggles'.

Precautions:

- If the pain persists or gets worse, be sure to get it checked out by a medical professional.
- NB Backwards steps may cause difficulties for those with balance issues, i.e., Parkinson's disease.

Playing With Routine: Dancing With Life

Routine makes the day easier, and for children with special needs, these routines are crucial while also incredibly challenging to master and remember.

Whether it's a morning routine, after-school routine, or bedtime routine, these steps can become mundane.

When we infuse play, music, and movement into them we make this long learning process more memorable, more impactful, and more enjoyable for everyone involved.

Make these parts of the day valued memories rather than mundane and repetitive times that both of you dread. Participate and play through these moments, raise the stakes, get creative, have fun!

Routines are important, so set yourself up for success! Here are some tips:

- Warning time – always prepare an individual for what's coming/what is going to be expected.
- Set a timer or have a cue (transition music, funny saying, playful prompt).
- For more independence have visuals (social stories, routine strips, PECS?).
- Break down immediate steps (first, then, next).
- Give yourself achievable choices when you can.

And if you are working with a group rather than an individual:

- Ask what kind of mood you are in (use emojis, energy-level metaphors in XX).
- Ask what kind of image, play mood you want your routine to take.

Once all your building blocks are in place, be spontaneous and bring it to life!

Chapter 19

Avoiding New Niggles

Preparing The Body For Action

Full-Body Breathing

Having taken several workshops and short courses on breathing and realising the debt they all owe to Eastern practices,[1] I have found a simplified combination of them that works well. I call it 'Full-Body Breathing' because it 'images' the entire body in inhaling and exhaling.

- On each inhalation, imagine that the air is entering the body simultaneously from the toes, the fingertips, the head, as well as through the nose.
- Image the air proceeding along the limbs and through the entire torso – shoulders and pelvis, through the head and neck – into the lungs, belly, and diaphragm.
- On the exhale, the air is expelled in reverse, all through the body and out the limbs and head, as well as the lungs and nose.
- Note: when areas are sore, stiff, or injured, image breathing especially from all parts of the body into the affected area and 'feel it' fill with flowing air. It cuts pain and improves circulation to and through the area.

Tip: it takes practice to be able to do all the imaging simultaneously, but it is worth the time and effort.

Precaution: be careful not to lift the shoulders when inhaling. Shoulders stay down – as if anchored or connected to the pelvis as the air enters lungs and engages the diaphragm.

Benefits: when we switch from 'regular' to full-body breathing, our focus immediately switches from scattered time, energy, and emotions caused by external conditions to the internal task of *imaging* our breathing, thus centring ourselves.

- It instantly dispels physical, emotional, and emotional tension.
- It slows down breathing and makes it deep, even, and regular.
- It eliminates shallow or irregular breathing patterns.

DOI: 10.4324/9780429439803-26

- It can help induce meditation, relaxation, and even sleep.
- It helps reduce blood pressure.
- Because breathing engages the diaphragm, it creates more effective oxygen flow throughout the body, thereby improving energy output.

Centring: Inner Listening, Re-Setting From The Toes Up

This exercise is about inner 'listening', starting literally from the ground up – with our feet.

While I (GMF) refer to it as 'listening', it can also be referred to as 'seeing', or 'feeling' internally, or as all three. An important preparation for any movement session, centring is also excellent anytime during the day when we need a sure, quick emotional, mental and/or physical focus, or to expel excess tension.

- Think of yourself as a tree: movement comes directly from the ankles while the rest of the body stays straight (i.e., no bending at the waist, neck, or upper back).
- Stand tall, straight, with knees and shoulders relaxed.
- Feet are pointing straight ahead and are about shoulder-width apart.
- Gently shut, or semi-shut, your eyes and remember to breathe evenly and deeply.
- Make very small, slow, smooth movements so you can 'listen' how the muscles in your feet and throughout your entire body alter as your balance changes – even slightly.
- Start to rock very slightly and gently forward and back, but stay in balance: no bending at the waist, feet firmly on floor.
- Concentrate your inner hearing, seeing, feeling into the soles of your feet.
- Be aware of the continuous, surprising, adapting of muscles and tendons throughout your body as it moves above your feet.
- After a few repetitions of swaying forward and back, find your 'centre point' where your body is most relaxed and where the fewest muscles are in play. Remember this centre point.
- Now repeat this 'listening' from side to side, again *impulsing* from ankles, and without bending at the waist; do a few repetitions, then find and return to your centre.
- Repeat, but doing small circles, then circles of eight first in one direction and then the other.

Tips:

- This activity works best in bare or stockinged feet.
- Centring creates such a complete sense of 'grounding' and calm that I (GMF) always suggest that you follow it with a 'shake-out' to get energy moving throughout your body again.

Make sure:

- When moving backward, forward, and side to side, keep your movement small enough that you keep your feet on the floor at all times, with no lifting of toes or heels.
- Be careful do not hold your breath.
- Again, thinking of yourself as a tree will help anchor the idea that all swaying movement initiates from the *ankles* only.

Precautions: if balance is an issue or if there is any danger of vertigo, allow tips of fingers on one hand to rest gently on the back of a chair, counter, or some similar object while doing this activity.

Benefits:

- It increases awareness of your balance points, posture and breathing.
- It counteracts feeling overwhelmed, tense, emotionally out of control, scattered, stressed.
- It will help slow down breathing, heartbeat, lower blood pressure
- It allows the mind and emotions to focus
- It creates a feeling of being 'grounded'

Shake-Outs

Many times during the day we find ourselves falling into *bad habits*, such as shallow breathing, holding our breath, or accumulating tension in shoulders, head, neck, etc. This exercise offers a two-second, effective way of 're-setting' – either increasing lagging energy or expelling excess energy, as well as re-establishing healthy breathing patterns.

- Stand comfortably, feet shoulder-width apart.
- Via negativa (see tips below): start by doing an exaggerated *inhale* and *hold your breath…*
- Still holding your breath, do a vigorous 'shake-out' – and don't keep your feet glued to the floor, but bounce or 'jog' on the spot while shaking limbs.
- After a count of one second, keep shaking-out, but *exhale* and release your voice very loudly and deliberately.
- Be aware of what happens as you exhale breath and voice: you should feel the tension literally slide out of your body, through your arms, head, legs, and feet.

Tips:

- 'Via negativa' is a term my teacher, Lecoq, used frequently: while learning a new exercise, you first deliberately do the movement 'the wrong way' so the body can recognise the difference from then on.

- Always do shake-outs after centring to reboot energy throughout the body.

Precautions: if you cannot jog on the spot or at least bounce during shake-out, you may also do it sitting on a chair or stool.

Benefits:

- Increases energy if you are feeling depleted
- Helps expel excess physical, mental, or emotional energy, tension, or anxiety
- Helps re-establish healthy breathing patterns.

Getting Out Of A Chair Safely

People often get out of a chair in ways that place stress on their knees or create a sharp rise in blood pressure that puts additional stress on their hearts and lungs. Here is a simple way of getting in and out of any chair in a safe and relatively stress-free way.

- Sit in *Fingers Dripping Water* position, ideally on the front third of the chair

  a Turn your palms to face behind you.

- Keeping your feet hip-width apart

  a Slide your right foot forward, stopping when its heel is level with the big toe of the left foot.

- Keeping your right foot pointing forward

  a Turn your left foot out 45 degrees away from your right foot.

- Inhale

  a Swing your hands up in front of body, stopping when at your eye-brow level.

- Keep your palms facing downwards, as if resting on a bar.
- Exhale

  a Float your hands back to *Fingers Dripping Water*

- Repeat twice
- On the *third inhalation*

  a As you swing your arms upwards, *stand up.*

- Exhale.

Make sure:

- The big toe of your front foot points in the same direction as your nose
- Your heels are about hip-width apart
- The big toe of your back foot points *away* from your front foot
- You inhale as you swing your arms upwards and stand up.

Precautions: use extreme care if your balance is unsteady or you use a walker to move around.

Benefits:

- Prevents rapid elevation in blood pressure
- Reduces strain on knees and abdominal muscles.

Helping Others Get Out Of A Chair

More and more people are looking after aged and sick relatives. Many end up helping their loved one stand up and remove themselves from the chair on which they are sitting. Here is a simple way to help do this without injuring yourself in the process.[2]

- Stand facing your loved one in *Bow Stance*[3] so that your right foot is as close as possible to the person who is seated comfortably on a chair.
- Breathing *in*
    - Release your hips and knees so that your back is straight and your hips back and arms are moving forward.
- Breathing *out*
    - Release your hips and knees so that your back is straight and your chest is slightly in front of your hips.
- Your loved one places each of their arms on the inside of your arms, if they can do so, grabbing or holding as close to your elbow as possible.
- Place your hands securely on the back of your loved one's upper arm, ideally just above each of their elbows – effectively cradling and securing their elbow.
- Inhale
- Exhale
    - Move your hips forward, simultaneously straightening your knees while lifting your loved one in an up and forward direction, towards the caregiver.

Precaution: if the resident is very heavy or has significant mobility restrictions, then a second person may be needed to balance the movement from behind.

The Wheelbarrow: How To Safely Lift A Heavy Object Up From The Floor

This exercise uses the same biodynamic motion that is used for working with a wheelbarrow.

- Begin in *Bow Stance*
  - a Stand in *Wu Chi*
  - b Slide right foot forward until heel is level with toes of left foot
  - c Pivoting on left heel, turn the left heel outward 45 degrees.
- Inhale
  - a Release your hips and knees so that your back is straight, and your chest is slightly in front of your hips.
- Exhale
  - a Hips move backward while chest leans forward; keep your back straight
  - b Place hands on the object.
- Inhale
  - a Grasp the object
  - b Move your hips forward while straightening your knees
    - Raise the object to waist level
    - Note: the heavier the object, the closer it should be held to the body.
- Exhale.

Lateral Mobility: 360-Degree Fitness

A fit, elderly friend broke a hip when she fell sideways … onto grass. When she protested that she rode a stationary bike "thirty minutes daily", her doctor asked, "Okay, but what do you do to keep your lateral muscles strong and responsive?"

Think of the space around you as circular, like the face of a clock. We usually work on a forward axis – from the centre to twelve o'clock … perhaps veering occasionally to eleven or one but ignoring backward to six o'clock or sideways to three or nine o'clock.

Here are two short, easy, and effective exercises to play with anytime during the day.

Lateral Mobility: Side-Stepping Over Logs

- As the title suggests, imagine you are surrounded by logs whose dimensions are wide and high.

- Lift your right leg as high as possible as you step sideways over the log to your right, so you end up straddling the log
- Shift your weight to your right side and lift your left leg over the log so you are once again standing, feet together.
- Repeat the action to the left.
- Do either one step in each direction, or do a series to one side, then reverse.
- Note: as you improve, the width and height of logs will increase.
- Remembering the space on the floor around you as a clock face, try stepping over logs at two, four, six, eight, and ten o'clock.

Tips:

- Lift the leg using glut and outer thigh muscles, not just torso. Try to keep torso upright.
- To avoid balance issues, gently hold onto counter or back of a steady chair while you accustom yourself to the exercises.

Lateral Mobility: Jack-Knives

- The image of a jack-knife is the guide for this lateral mobility activity.
- The supporting leg is like the knife blade that is opened while the entire rest of the jack-knife leans over.
- In this activity, the entire torso and the lifting leg stay in a straight line – like the body of a jack-knife. When the moving leg is lifted, the torso leans over in perfect line with it.

Tips:

- Compare the role of the torso in Side-Stepping Over Logs, where the emphasis is on lifting the moving leg while keeping the torso as upright as possible; in Jack-Knives, the lifting leg and the torso lean simultaneously in a perfectly straight line.
- To avoid balance issues, gently hold onto a counter or back of a steady chair while you accustom yourself to the exercises.

Benefits of Side-Stepping Over Logs and Jack-Knives:

- Both activities increase:

  a Strength and control of leg and torso muscles
  b 360-degree reflexes – the ability to react with more speed and agility
  c Confidence and ease of movement.

Feather Drawing: Joint Relaxers and Mobilisers

During a long, acute bout of plantar fasciitis, after a Feldenkrais class on foot and ankle mobility with practitioner Fariya Doctor, I (GMF) was shocked by the muscle tension it released – and how much it alleviated the pain in my foot and arch.

- All exercises referred to as 'feather drawing' are to be done *very gently*, without any strain in the effort – as the title suggests, as if being drawn by a feather.
- These exercises can be done standing or sitting.

Feather Circles: Heel/Ankle

- If standing have feet close together, knees relaxed (not bent, not locked straight)
- If in a chair, sit on the front third of the chair so feet are resting flat on floor, not too far apart but not touching.
- Shift weight to left side, and while keeping balls of right foot lightly on the floor, lift right heel and draw several large clockwise feather circles; place right foot back on floor and switch to left foot heel circles.
- Repeat heel feather circles but going in counter-clockwise direction. Balls of foot may lift slightly during counter-clockwise circles.
- If sitting, try doing heel circles with both feet simultaneously.

Feather Fans: Full Foot/Ankle

- If standing, have your feet close together, knees relaxed (not bent, not locked straight).
- If in a chair, sit on the front third of the chair so feet are resting flat on floor, not too far apart but not touching.
- Shift weight to left side and keep right heel on floor as the rest of the foot lifts very slightly so it can pivot gently from right to left, like a fan, just barely touching the floor surface. Especially if done standing, side-to-side fan-like movement may extend to knee and hip.
- Place right foot back on floor and switch to left foot/ankle fans.
- If sitting, try doing foot/ankle side-to-side fans with both feet simultaneously.

Feather Circles, Feather Fans: Other Joints

With a bit of imagination, you can replicate and adapt the Feather Circles and Feather Fans movements to any major joints. If circular or fan movements are done with a 'feather' touch, any joint should immediately feel lighter, less tense, or painful, and with more ease of movement.

Hands And Wrists

- Place your hands on a table, desk, or counter
- Repeat Feather Circles and Feather Fan movements just as you did with feet and ankles:

  a the heels of your hand = heels of your feet.
  b your wrists = your ankles.
  c your fingertips = your toes and balls of the feet.

Shoulders, Elbows, Hips

- Feather Circles: each of the abovementioned joints can do circles.
- Feather Fans: experiment moving each of these joints 'back and forth', in a fan-like movement. If you maintain the 'feather' touch, you should feel the instant relief of released tension.

Tips for all Feather Drawing exercises:

- Remember to breathe normally – full-body breathing is best – during exercises.
- If balance is an issue, hold on to the back of a chair or countertop.
- Be sure you are not tensing other parts of the body while doing the Feather movements.

Benefits:

- Increases blood circulation
- Releases muscle tension
- Increases mobility in all joints being 'feather moved'.
- Allows feet and ankles to recognise and respond to underfoot stimuli (such as uneven surfaces, objects, or textures underfoot that may cause problems).

Notes

1 See chapter 13, 'Essential Eastern Exercises'.
2 The directions are written for family members providing home care but apply equally well if you are a care giver working in any assisted living, aged care, long-term care, or nursing home facility.
3 Stand in *Wu Chi*. Slide your right foot forward until your heel is level with toes of your left foot. Pivot on your left heel and turn your left heel outward 45 degrees away from your right foot.

Chapter 20

Exploring Your Body And Space

First Steps: The Eight Points of Balance/Travel

Imagine you are standing at the centre of an analogue clock.

- Begin in *Standing Post* position, with both arms loosely by your sides.
- On an in-breath, with your eyes closed, raise one arm in the direction of your body's movement

    a Arm is raised from the side of the body slowly
    b The hand drags along the torso
    c Hand flips to palm facing up and begins to reach out once it hits the shoulder area, your first finger leading in a grand pointing gesture.

- Without moving your feet, slowly *lean* until your body starts to tip.
- Continue as far as you can until you fall and are required to take one step only.

Explore all eight basic directions of travel:

1 Straight back – six o'clock
2 Back to the right corner
3 Straight to the right side – three o'clock
4 Forward to the right corner
5 Straight forward – 12 noon
6 Forward to the left corner
7 Straight to the left – nine o'clock
8 Back to the left corner.

Between each movement return to centre to the *Standing Post* position.

Kinesphere – For One

Kinesphere describes the space around your body, no matter where you are standing, and the potential range of gestures available to you, no matter

DOI: 10.4324/9780429439803-27

where you are positioned in a space. You can explore this space around you without travelling or moving your feet off the spot on which you are standing.

This exercise allows you to explore how far you can extend different parts of your body.

It allows you to explore your kinesphere in interesting ways by varying the speed and/or range, and/or intent of any movement without moving your feet off the spot on which you are standing

If you like, you can play soft slow rhythmic music during this exercise.

- Stand anywhere with your feet hip-width apart and your knees relaxed.
- Imagine you are encased in a semi-permeable, breathable membrane.
- This membrane responds like a malleable plastic responds to pressure.
- Initially it is hard to move and requires effort – *however*, the more you move the softer the membrane becomes.

Slowly move *isolated* individual elements of your body:

- Start by focusing on your fingers, then, one at a time:

  a Hands
  b Arms
  c Torso
  d Legs
  e Feet
  f Toes.

- Start to combine

  a Two body elements
  b Three body elements
  c Any elements you want.

Tips:

- Throughout this process imagine *breathing into* your joints, especially the 'articulating' joints – i.e. those in your elbows, knees, shoulders, etc.
- Once you get comfortable with this exercise you can try experimenting with:

  a Different styles of music as a stimulus for your movement
  b Taking a travel step – i.e., moving your position in the room by one step.

Impulsing: Directing Energy

The impulse and drive for any movement we make with our bodies does not always come from the torso area or shoulders, but rather from the exact area of the body part about to move. Imagine that the specific body part to move seems to be pushed in a direction by its own jet engines or pulled up by puppet strings. For example:

- Action: lift your arm, palm facing down.
- Ask yourself: where does the 'drive' come from? Is it from the shoulder? Does your arm feel somewhat heavy and awkward? If it does, then lower arm.
- Shifting the impulse: lift, then lower your arm, but on the lift, image/imagine that:

  a You have a little jet engine under the palm of the hand that thrusts the arm upward
  b Your arm is lifted by a puppet string attached to the top of your moving hand.

- Be aware of how different the movement feels if the impulse comes from the hand itself, rather than from the shoulder.
- Try the idea of pushing with jets and/or lifting with puppet strings using different joints or body parts, such as:

  a The knee, heel, or top of foot arch for stepping, running, climbing, kicking (heel)
  b Elbows or shoulders.

Tips:

- Be aware of the difference in the 'quality' of the movement when jets or strings are used as the image source. For example, for pushing, kicking, hitting, etc., jets are excellent for strength, drive, and accuracy; for ease, fluidity and efficacy of movement, strings work best.
- For more complex actions, such as climbing stairs, lifting, manoeuvring obstacles, etc., try shifting impulse and image from one body part to another, depending on what is needed to complete the action.
- For greatest mobility, ease, and fluid movements, always think of extending the limbs away from the body as you execute a movement, rather than letting them 'fall back into the body'.

Benefits:

- Having the impulse originate from specific body parts should result in more clarity, precision, control, and ease of movement. Examples: when walking on ice or precarious surfaces; or needing sudden, fast, and targeted strong responses (pushing, catching, stopping, jabbing, swatting, etc.)

- Directed impulses create economy of movement and help avoid over-straining or stressing shoulders, neck, knees, or hip flexors.
- Puppet string impulses allow movement to be executed with grace, ease, and flow.

Chapter 21

Exploring Movement Vocabulary

Painting The Floor – For One

- Imagine you are an artist creating a painting on the floor
  - a The floor is your canvas
  - b Your feet are your paint brushes.
  - c As you move your feet paint the canvas.
- Explore moving your feet in
  - a Straight lines
  - b Circles
  - c Spirals
  - d Figures of eight.
  - e Combinations of circles, straight lines, and spirals
  - f Jumps
    - Straight up
    - Up and over
    - Imagine a small bench that needs clearing.
- Dab paint on the canvas
  - a Lightly
  - b Heavily.
- Caress the canvas in different ways.
- Use any other 'brush stroke' you can think of!

Play music with a variety of tempos and rhythms and styles. Here, in no particular order, are some pieces of music I have used a lot:

a Scatterlings Of Africa – Juluka
b Bach's Goldberg Variations – Glenn Gould
c Chinese folk tunes
d Strut – Sheena Easton

DOI: 10.4324/9780429439803-28

e Bolero – Ravel
f Objection (Tango) – Shakira
g La Estempe Reale (Spanish Court Dance) – Albion Band
h Walk This Way – Aerosmith
i Variations On My Lady Carey's Dompe – John Renbourne
j On The Floor – J-Lo
k Lazarus Heart – Sting
l Reels Part II – My Love Is In America (Titanic) – Bad Haggis

After practising this exercise a few times, try to imagine how the music might make you move before playing it. What colours and brush strokes you will use, what shapes you might make.

Take time between each piece of music to write about the experience – how you felt, words suggested, etc.

Note to group leaders: this is a great activity to use with groups.

Dance As If No One Is Watching

Everything Dances!

All living organisms dance. Human beings are no exception. We are constantly pursuing movements which have rhythm and repetition – loading a dishwasher, walking to work, making coffee … – that can be subdivided into movement themes or phrases. In fact, several modern choreographers have built on these natural movement sequences to create dances that audiences pay money to watch.

- Put music on and dance freely without inhibition, shyness, or any worry about 'what you look like'

  a If you want, you can do this sitting on a chair.

- Play a selection of any music you want

  a Pop
  b Soft jazz
  c Techno
  d Rock and roll
  e A random selection.

- Challenge yourself

  a Move with the rhythm of the music
  b Move against the rhythm of the music

c Isolate elements of your body and move

- Only your arms
- Only your feet.

d Freeze like a statue

- On a natural pause
- Anywhere in the 'track' for a count of 3–5 in your head.

Note to group leaders: this is a great activity to use with groups. You can ask the group to bring their own music selections with them to the dance/movement sessions. If you have an established group, make different participants responsible for the music selection each session.

Chapter 22

Reducing Stress

Breathe And 'Mumble'

One way of making sure you are breathing correctly, without holding your breath, as well as engaging your muscles smoothly while moving, is to mumble, hum, sing, talk, or recite a poem. The quality of your 'mumble' tells you how well you are moving and breathing and can help you correct any poor habits.

- Just *before* you begin moving, start quietly 'mumbling' ("mumble, mumble" works as a text) and continue until you finish the movement.
- Be aware of how your breath sounds: you should be able to carry on a conversation without others being aware that you are exercising.
- If you are grunting, stop-starting, or changing your pitch, it means that you are pushing your muscles and breathing unevenly in response, rather than having muscles work smoothly *with the breath.*
- Remember you are to *exhale* during the *effort part* of the movement in order to support your muscle effort.
- Go back to the moments in the exercise when the mumble-glitch happens. Start mumbling (exhaling) and engage your muscles before the problem point and practise having your muscles smoothly respond to the exercise so you are exhaling and mumbling smoothly before, during, and after the problem point. Repeat until it becomes natural and easy.

Benefits:

- Holding our breath or breathing irregularly during exercises actually makes the movements harder to do, tends to *increase* accumulated tension, causes our blood pressure to rise, and can leave us out of breath.
- The advantage of mumbling is that you can hear yourself – you don't need someone directing you.
- As well, the *quality* of the mumble tells you if your muscles and your breathing are harmonious, or if you are retaining tension and adding to

DOI: 10.4324/9780429439803-29

stress by a) pushing too hard with your muscles, and b) catching your breath, which will make the mumbles sound 'stumbly' and jagged.

Consonant Karate

- Shape your hands into a karate knife hand (karate chop).
- Now chop the air with your hands and stamp your feet.
- While making these motions

  a Exhale forcefully making the sound of a hard consonant, *c, t, d*, or *g*.

    - The sounds *f, b*, and *sh* may also be used.

Note to group leaders: this is a great activity to use with groups. The game can be converted to a rhythmic tribal dance by positioning the group in two well-spaced lines facing one another. These lines can then move together and apart, stamping, and exhaling consonant sounds.

Care should be taken to emphasise that this is a non-contact dance.

Temper Tantrums

Temper Tantrums is the perfect answer for those times when we just have to release or even avoid extra stress, pent-up anxieties, or those body, mind, and emotion knots! They are highly adaptable to personal needs and contexts and make a great individual or group activity. And you can add your own text! They are particularly freeing if you begin with negativity and proceed to positive, wildly extravagant, and enjoyable promises of self-empowerment.

- Temper Tantrums can be done by having participants walking in a large circle or by staying in one spot, sitting in chairs, or even lying on the floor.
- Accompany all movements with text or loud sounds.
- Start with 'angry' actions and text with negative phrases and progress to positive ones. Note: going from positive to negative makes life afterwards seem less possible.
- Start with rhythmic stomps on floor if sitting in chair, or marching or rocking body and stomping fists and feet if lying down. Text: on the beat, say things like "No, I won't" or "I don't want to".
- Advance to strutting with hips and shoulders twisting, nose petulantly in the air, and a text like "Maybe yes and maybe no".
- Punch in front and up into the air as you do large advancing lunge-like steps or lean forward or look up into the air if in chairs; bang feet (gently on floor) during punches if lying down … with text such as "No, I won't" or "Go away" or "No waaayyyy".

- Then, keep large steps (lunges) or start skipping while altering from anger punches to fun-defiant 'flick-slaps' of the hands with "Yes, I will" or "I can if I want" or "You can't stop me!"
- Finish off with exuberant hops and jumps (if possible), or simply quick steps, while joyfully collecting and tossing both hands in the air as if throwing armfuls of petals into the sky, with "Yes, I can!" or "I'm ready" or "Just watch me!" – people will soon want to create their own phrases with the movements.
- Finalise activities with joyous, unanimous loud 'yeeeaaaayyy!' victory calls and energetic clapping (and leaps if you can and wish to!).

Tip: if working in groups, make sure that participants keep enough distance from each other to be able to walk, sit, or lie down without hitting each other.

Precautions:

- Words and text can be altered at will but avoid 'charged' words or phrases – 'gibberish'[1] is a perfect solution. It can be difficult at the beginning but becomes easier.
- Likewise, if there are any possible antagonisms in group, be sure that those involved are not working near each other and be prepared to use 'freeze' if necessary.
- In cases where there are known antagonisms, the sitting in chairs or lying down versions are preferable.

Benefits:

- Excellent for reducing stress, anxiety, and negative feelings.
- Very good for community building and creating a fun and safe environment.
- Combines voice, breathing, movement, mind, and emotions into one activity.
- Helps re-boot focus.

Note

1 Gibberish is simply 'pretend talking', using sounds that are 'spoken' and may sound like words, but are just strings of imaginary utterings.

Part VII

Working With Groups

In this extended section, the authors change focus to include suggestions and ideas for individuals running classes and workshops for others who wish to do the same. They also provide exercises and approaches to employ in working with different groups.

DOI: 10.4324/9780429439803-30

Chapter 23

Leading Movement Workshops And Classes

Helping Others Change Their Story

Planning and Leading Movement Workshops: An Introduction

Most of the focus of this book is on taking charge of our own lives. In this section we change focus to include suggestions and ideas for those of you who, in addition to engaging in healthy movement practices in your own daily life, are also running classes and workshops for others who wish to do the same.

Leadership As Story-Zoom

A well-organised and executed class or workshop is much the same as a good story well read. In many ways, the leader of a class or workshop is the narrator of the story, improvising and developing while doing the telling.

As with a story, as leader you must define your central theme when planning a workshop for a group. Coming up with a title for the session, even if it is just one class in a long semester, often helps clarify what your story is about. And remember, clarity of mind is important as you can only tell one story at a time!

Each new story is created via careful planning and consideration of unique elements, the so-called dramatic questions: Who? Where? When? Why? The so-called 'given circumstances' that help create the what and why of the story.

Who Am I? What Are My Skill Sets?

The Medium May Be The Message, But The Individual Is The Method

Marshall McLuhan once said the "Medium is the Message"[1]; however, in our conversations with the late Professor Richard Courtney, he maintained that rather than follow a fixed script, each individual teacher must make their skill sets the vehicle by which they teach any class or workshop.

Successful workshops can involve different approaches, and these in large part depend on the nature of the leader. Some leaders need a tightly organised

DOI: 10.4324/9780429439803-31

checklist, others need to run each session off the cuff and improvise the whole thing. While many leaders will need something between those two. The important thing is to learn about yourself as a workshop leader and find what works best for you; start by answering the question, "Who am I?"

I (BW) have been training teachers and workshop leaders since 1973. My own leadership style has been strongly influenced by three very different individuals. Each had their own way of leading workshops because their strengths were very different.

a Bert Amies: a theatre director who took a very cerebral, quiet, and analytical approach. Who asked questions of the participants in such a way that they thought they had found the answers for themselves. When in fact Bert was 'seeding' these through each activity.
b Yon: a musical conductor, dancer, and poet who was very expressive. He sang and danced through everything. More impressive than this was his economy of activity. He could use the same four activities for exploration of many different ideas and adapt the same activity for all ages and abilities.
c George Major: a dancer, choreographer, and theatre director who was always blunt and challenging! It didn't matter whether he was addressing an ex-principal dancer from a major dance company, a young student, or a person who used a wheelchair, he would be constantly challenging participants who he thought were on auto pilot, calling it in, with "TATATA! You're boring me, do something different."

One other person who also influenced me was David Booth, who would speak so quietly you had to lean in to hear him – leading your interest.

Given Circumstances

- *Who?*
  a Who are you?
    - What are your strengths as a workshop leader?
    - What is your preferred leadership style?

  b Who are your participants?
    - What are their strengths?
    - Who is shy and will need extra encouragement?
    - Who among them are the natural leaders?
- *When?*
  a Time of day?
  b Duration?

- *Where?*

  a Does the room have:

    - Natural light?
    - A dance floor/carpet?

- *Why?*

  a What is the reason for this session?

- *What?*

  a What story do you wish to tell?
  b What's the topic of your workshop?
  c What are your goals/objectives?
  d What do you hope to accomplish by the end of this session?

- *How?*

  a How do you speak to the group?

    - Pitch/pace/tone?
    - Humour?
    - Song?

  b How do you deliver explanations?

    - How much detail?
    - Let them learn as they go?
    - How do you intend to deal with unplanned events?

  c How will you deal with:

    - Latecomers
    - People dressed inappropriately (in suits!)
    - Unacceptable or offensive behaviours or language?

  d Do you plan for your group?

    - Given all the information you have, how can you best achieve your goals?
    - What activities will best match your strengths with the perceived needs of your group and their abilities?
    - How much structure do you need to provide for the group so they can actively engage in these activities?

The Story Arc

- Each story arc is comprised of and supported by the moments/activities (mini arcs) in that session.

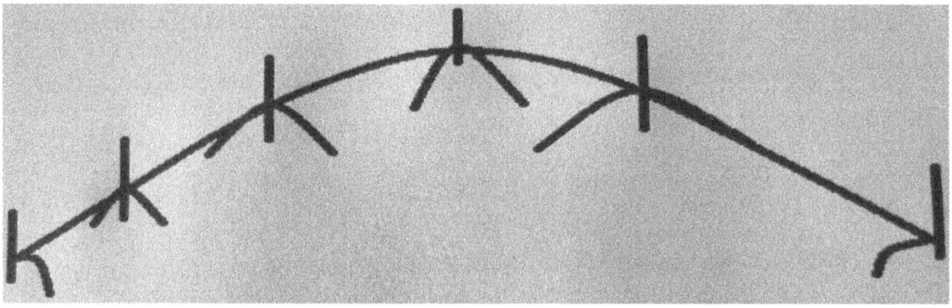

Figure 23.1 Story Arc

- Each mini arc can be as steep (quick) or drawn out (longer time allotted) as needed.
- The vertical line represents the peak of the activity that is connected back to the overall arc (class/workshop learning goals).

Arc Shape Elements

- *Framing*: how to present learning
- *Phrasing*: shape of the workshop arc and mini arcs – how you present them, what you include. They can be:

  a Standard
  b Sharp peak
  c Drawn out.

- *Pacing*: how much time getting info from/about the group at the beginning?

  a How much time do you allow them to digest each activity?

- *Interacting*: do you give every participant the exact same opportunity? Or do you use volunteers to demonstrate activities, etc.?

  a Discussion time: do you direct the questions at people or ask openly? Or do you ask at the end of each activity or at end of workshop?

- *Learning*: the objective of the workshop!

  a Cannot plan long-term outcomes without multiple workshops
  b Focus learning on what you can control, the present workshop.

Note

1 M. McLuhan (1964), *Understanding Media: The Extensions of Man* (New York: McGraw-Hill).

Chapter 24

Introducing Dance-Movement To 'Non-Dancers'

> I've always slightly regretted that I'm not a dancer.[1]

As we discussed earlier in this book, everything involves dance. Making breakfast, sweeping the floor are sequences of movements repeated in ritualistic fashion that may be considered a dance. Everyday activities and everyday movements are often the framework and vocabulary used by choreographers to create dance performances. Yet most people either underrate their capabilities ("I am not a dancer") or overate them – most recently, on Tik Tok. Either way, as Alan Cummins has noted, "the strict expectation that a dancer is someone with a particular technique and physique only stymies the art form".[2]

In 1980 I (BW) was 'head-hunted' straight out of college to work for LUDUS Dance-in-Education company. As a mature student, I had just completed a BA (Hons) in Creative Arts with what Americans would probably call a double major in drama and creative writing and a minor in dance. I should add this was my second kick at the can as I had already completed studies in psychology and education.

I was hired as educational researcher/deputy director of the Special Schools Project, 'Learning Through Dance'.[3] In addition to my responsibilities to the project,[4] I also ran a weekly dance-movement class, Dance For the Non-Dancer (DFND). The promotional materials for the class was as follows:

> *Dance For The Non-Dancer* provides a fun, flexible and improvisational approach to creative movement and dance, which allows you to explore and enjoy the movement of your body. The program presents simple games and exercises drawn from a variety of movement and dance styles that are easy to participate in and enjoyable.
>
> Whether you have a little or a lot of dance/movement training or simply enjoy dancing in the comfort of your living room: *Dance For The Non-Dancer* is designed to provide an experience that can be enjoyed by anyone.

DOI: 10.4324/9780429439803-32

The concept was simple. At the time, the professional dancers of LUDUS ran several evening technique classes in ballet, contemporary, etc., for the community; DFND was to be a 'pre-technique' class. The hope was that by having experienced and enjoyed this class, students would go on to take one or more of the technique classes.

Some people did do this, but many more simply came to enjoy the freedom of what Peter Slade referred to as *natural* dance,[5] the ability to allow ourselves to simply enjoy moving. The class was mainly dance-movement games, free-form movement to music (both individual and group) and Contact Improvisation/Contact Release – something in which I was relatively expert.

In the beginning the class was a broad mix of people who had a little dance experience and those who had none. After a few sessions, people discovered that in this class people had fun and found camaraderie and community. Not only did the class meet regularly once a week but I also organised weekend retreats for participants.

The most important point for me as a teacher of 'non-dancers' was *never* to criticise an individual's form or technique[6] but rather to gently encourage and challenge everyone within the limits of their own movement vocabulary and flexibility. This approach had been very much honed and amplified working in the schools as part of the Special Schools Project, where my task was to work with students with severe physical and intellectual challenges in their attempts to master any movement task.

Word of mouth spread, and by the last few sessions I found that in addition to my usual participants the class included experienced dancers who wanted a break from the rigours of technique.[7] Any dancer who was in town would drop in and take a DFND class. When I moved to Canada, I handed over the running of my class to a former principal dancer from the Stuttgart Ballet who had enjoyed the class so much he decided to stay in Lancaster.

Lessons Learned From DFND

The lessons I learned from my work with LUDUS and especially from teaching DFND classes stayed with me throughout my professional life. Throughout my 35-year academic career no matter what other classes I taught, I always enjoyed teaching the introductory movement classes.

The students in my classes were always a mixed bunch – from those individuals who had been dancing since they were three to those who had never had a formal movement class in their life. My greatest joy was to see individuals who were convinced they had two wooden left feet discovering freedom of movement and exploring the expressiveness of their body through the movement vocabulary and structures I provided them in the classes.

I came to realise that to help 'non-dancers' be and feel 'successful'– to feel the joy of simply moving – in addition to not criticising but encouraging and challenging, the tasks and activities provided needed to:

- Be attainable
- Follow the KISS (Keep It Simple Stupid) principle
  a Be broken down into very simple 'bite size' pieces.
- Follow the 'Bach' principle
  a Introduction of each new activity should build slowly in layers upon the one(s) that precede it – like a Bach fugue.

Using these simple rules as a guide I pride myself that former students, many of whom were 'non-dancers', contact me on a regular basis to tell how much they cherish the experiences gained through the movement classes and what the classes have meant to their life.

Notes

1 L. Winship (2022), www.theguardian.com/stage/2022/aug/03/alan-cumming-youd-be-shocked-by-the-messages-miriam-margolyes-and-i-leave-each-other?CMP=Share_iOSApp_Other
2 L. Winship (2022), www.theguardian.com/stage/2022/aug/03/alan-cumming-youd-be-shocked-by-the-messages-miriam-margolyes-and-i-leave-each-other?CMP=Share_iOSApp_Other
3 The Special Schools Project was an ambitious project carried out in 1980–82 with support and funding from three education authorities, The Schools Council, The Calouste Gulbenkian Foundation, and The Arts Council of Great Britain, plus numerous other arts and educational bodies. The project involved nearly thirty special schools catering for over 2,000 children with a wide range of physical, intellectual, and emotional disabilities. It brought together a professional dance/theatre company with teachers, educational researchers, arts therapists, and special school children. The project raised the profile of the arts on the special education curriculum, trained teachers in the use of the arts with special children, and made many suggestions about the preparation, development, and presentation of professional theatre performances in special schools.
4 These included developing and writing educational materials to accompany the dance-theatre performance, *The Thunder Tree,* and delivering post-performance workshops for students and in-service training workshops for teachers.
5 In *Natural Dance* Peter Slade describes his philosophy of dance based on the individual style that belongs to each personality. He suggests liberating or encouraging natural improvised dance and developing this through polished improvisation to dance drama, and from dance drama to an advanced professional level of grace, beauty, and competence. he builds a bridge between improvisation and technique; he proposes dance can be enjoyed at every level, from the early childhood years to adult life; by those who are physically fit, by people living with a disability and by people in every kind of profession or occupation.
6 Unfortunately, all too often savage criticism is the hallmark of technique classes, something that anyone who has ever taken a dance technique class is painfully aware.
7 Something that is becoming more present in the 21st century are professional dancers who engage in Yoga, Pilates, pole dance, and acro-gymnastics in addition to their continuing rigorous training in dance technique.

Chapter 25

A Few Words On Adapting To The Needs Of Your Group

I am not my disability, I am me.[1]

When planning a workshop or lesson, it is easy to get carried away with an abstract idea. Words on a page which describes the arc of the story. However, it is never that simple! In his ground-breaking book, *The Empty Space*, the legendary theatre director Peter Brook talks of his first experience of directing a play, *Loves Labours Lost*, at Stratford. He pre-rehearsed the entrance to the play for the forty actors involved, using similar-sized folded cardboard models. He talks of how the next day the entrance itself was a mess, nothing like he planned. How he foolishly thought that an inanimate model can stand in for real human beings of different sizes, with different rhythms, movements, and emotions.

So, when planning always remember no two individuals, even *monozygotic twins*, are exactly the same. No two groups are the same, either. This makes planning difficult and may become more so if, even as an experienced leader, you fail to plan for each new group as if for the first time.

The simple rule is that each lesson/workshop plan should be tailored to the individual needs of the participants within your group. However, in the 21st century this often means planning for a group of individuals who:

- Identify on a broad spectrum of sexual identities.
  a This brings up linguistic challenges concerning, among other things, personal pronouns.
- Have grown up in a wide range of cultural, geographic, religious, and linguistic environments
  a This brings with it issues related to cultural, racial, religious, and ethnic sensitivities.
- Live with both visible and invisible disabilities
  a This brings planning challenges in terms of mobility, linguistic comprehension, and the ability to process ideas, commands, and thoughts.

DOI: 10.4324/9780429439803-33

There is no single or simple fool-proof solution to this conundrum. However, over the years I (BW) have developed some strategies to try to avoid major blunders.

- Even though anecdotal stories, case studies, and prior academic reports may be helpful, it must be remembered that they are filtered through the lens of other people's biases and expectations. So, while useful, prior information must be taken with a pinch of salt.
- Always try to interact with each person prior to starting the first session. Take time to ask if an individual has any restrictions or concerns of which you should be aware.
- In addition, try whenever possible to begin your first session by playing simple name game – e.g., This Is My Name.[2]

  a Not only does this provide information about each participant, it also helps build group cohesion.

Notes

1 Swann in Exley (1984).

2 Participants stand in a circle facing each other. Each person introduces themself by saying their first name and sharing some information about it – for example:

- The meaning of the name – e.g., Bernard means Heart of the Bear
- Who they were named after/for
- Why that name was chosen
- How they feel about their name
- Each person finishes by saying: "My name is …".

A more detailed version of this appears in B. Warren and P. Spitzer (2014), *Smiles Are Everywhere* (London/New York: Routledge).

Chapter 26

Zoom-Zoom: Digital Movement Classes/Workshops

The Covid pandemic came to test our resilience, creativity, intelligence, and common sense. Given that our society has been 'hooked on visuals' in almost all aspects of our lives since well before Covid, we might have expected that with the worldwide life disruptions it caused, we would have effortlessly slid into all things virtual. That didn't necessarily happen.

The tech companies did burst into action, providing ever-expanding platforms to invite us to communicate, to connect, if only virtually. However, in many ways that very early lockdown period caused many people, organisations, and endeavours to go into paralysis mode. It was as if we became as immobile and 'locked in' as the immutable screens being used to frame our faces and our (in)actions.[1]

Schools and school boards everywhere froze in 'pande-panic'. It was assumed we now most definitely had to 'sit still and be quiet' while teaching methods that slide backward into the most stultifying rote methods were encouraged as being utterly necessary.

The sense of paralysis spread quickly and questions of how to turn this sudden obstacle into an opportunity didn't get asked. The possibility of truly creative solutions didn't seem to come into enough minds. One drama teacher, forced to teach a post-secondary course online, told students that there would be no movement or interactive drama activities, since "how could you do movement or interact from the shoulders up?" Luckily, one student pointed out that his mom had been doing Yoga online since way before Covid.

For years, Ontario's dance and drama teachers had been working to include and retain dance and drama in the curriculum, but those in power assumed that, with Covid, these subjects would be impossible and, therefore, immediately expendable. However, that assumption had an opposite, invigorating effect!

Many of these teachers were not prepared to abandon such clearly visual art forms, especially if there was any chance of being able to use virtual platforms. They *did* look for creative solutions. One successful example came from the Ontario Secondary School DanceFest (OSSDF). Covid lockdown began just weeks before their annual festival, which had to be cancelled.[2] However, they re-scheduled it as a virtual event. Students from participating

DOI: 10.4324/9780429439803-34

schools sent in videos of their dances, which occurred in closets, backyards, abandoned lots, under tables – anywhere and everywhere. All dancers wore masks, whether dancing alone or in small groups.

Teaching Dance-Movement Therapy At A Distance

I (BW) had my first experience of teaching movement at a distance when in 1985 I helped develop a course, Introduction to Therapeutic Arts, for Okanagan College which was offered in part on-site and in part at a distance. This course was developed seven years before even dial-up internet was available commercially, and the internet and Wi-Fi as we know it in the 21st century not only did not exist but had not even been conceived of!

On two Saturdays I taught a dance-movement therapy component at a distance. I was in one studio while students in other studios spread throughout the Okanagan College network. There was a single camera in each studio and a noticeable time lapse between actions being completed and me seeing them. There was also a shaky element to all the images and the sound was out of synch with the image. Hardly a perfect or seamless way to teach anything, let alone movement! Suffice to say the course was not a success and was not repeated. However, the experience of teaching movement to students who were at a distance was both salutary and informative.

Teaching Movement To Chinese Students On WeChat

Following a highly successful four-day workshop, Foundations of Therapeutic Drama, that I taught in person in Shenzhen China, I was asked to do a follow-up workshop. Unfortunately, at this point Covid hit, making international travel impossible, so an in-person workshop was not an option. After long and convoluted negotiations, during which the sponsor for my workshops changed several times, in 2020 I finally agreed to offer a series of four online workshops, which would essentially be interactive graduate seminars.

Each workshop was designed to last two hours. The eight participants lived mainly in Shenzhen, but some lived in other locations in China. The workshops were all taught in English, but I also had a Chinese translator, Sami who was also my de facto graduate researcher/teaching assistant.

As the Chinese do not have easy access to most of the Western social media apps, the platform we used was WeChat.[3] It should be noted that this platform is not as flexible, stable, or user friendly as, say, Zoom.

The primary purpose of the workshops was to explore the therapeutic use of drama in psychological counselling. Because of my training and expertise and the problems of translation, I focused on family therapy and non-verbal interventions, always trying to be mindful of the cultural differences. It helped that I entered this process having already studied Chinese philosophy and culture, albeit as an outsider, for over fifty years.

After the first webinar, I was fascinated to realise how little the participants were aware of their own history and culture – at least as it had been explained to me during my lifelong study of Chinese martial and healing arts. So, I revised the content of the next workshop, and all subsequent ones, and used seated Qigong exercises and Taoist philosophy to 'package' and deliver Western drama/family therapy techniques related to dramatic imagination, transitional objects, personal stories, perspective, and inter-personal communication.[4]

I made short videos of each of the seated Qigong exercises and shared these with Sami before I taught them. Also, I met with Sami for 30–60 minutes before each webinar to make sure she understood both the exercises and the concepts I was endeavouring to teach. She was then able to help participants with the exercises and any questions they needed to ask. I should add that I used *very* simple Chinese words to teach the essence of each exercise and was even complimented on my pronunciation!

The workshop, unlike the in-service course, was a great success. Despite the problems of language and the limitations of the platform employed, it was possible to encourage a group of self-conscious individuals to engage in movement exercises from a great distance and in different time zones through a digital medium.

Notes

1 To offset this classroom, meeting, and general zoom-zombie effect, we (GMF) at DramaSound Projects developed a series of six short, simple routines called *ZOOM ZZZAPS*, meant as every-hour breaks to relax, re-engage and re-energise body, mind, and emotions. These can be accessed on YouTube through www.dramasoundprojects.com

2 From Laurel Brown, originator, and artistic director: "Live DANCEFEST events from 2003–2019 grew to affect approximately 500 students and dance educators annually. During the pandemic, OSSDF reinvented from a four-day live event to ten months of support for teachers with virtual dance workshops and dance artists' inspirational journeys shared every two weeks from September to June in 2021 and every month in 2022. This resulted in thirty workshops being created and shared with 10,895 students and teachers from 29 Ontario school boards."

3 WeChat is a Chinese platform like Facebook/Messenger and WhatsApp. It should be noted that Chinese social media activity is monitored by Chinese authorities.

4 Exercises shared:

Polishing The Table

- Imagine you have a soft glove on your hand and are carefully polishing a glass table.
- Coordinate circle movements with your breathing.

Rolling A Ball Of Energy

- Imagine you have a glass ball full of air/energy between your palms.

- Breathing in, slowly bend forward from your waist while at the same time moving this ball in a vertical circle.
- Breathing out, rock backwards, continuously moving ball in a large circle.

Parting The Clouds

- Imagine there are clouds above your head.
- Breathing in, move your hands up above your head and away from each other – moving the clouds apart and away from you.
- Breathing out, your hands circle down back to your lap.

Chapter 27

Movement And Community

For more than forty years I (BW) have been involved in developing and delivering healthy movement programmes within and for various communities. At the beginning of my career, as mentioned above in the Teaching Dance To Non-Dancers section, I ran dance-movement classes for people of all ages in schools, community centres, and seniors' centres. Later in my career I started to run martial arts and eastern healing programmes. Here I present a sample of some of the healthy movement programmes I designed and delivered.

Qigong For Healthy Adults[1]

In 1993, I met my current teacher Master George Ling Hu. At the time of meeting I had already been studying martial arts and Eastern healing approaches for 25 years and was teaching Qigong and Tai Chi as part of my academic Creative Movement classes at the University of Windsor. However, I learnt more from Master Hu in the first three hours than I had in the previous ten years of study and practice. This meeting was the point I consider my serious study of traditional Chinese health and martial arts began.

It was not long after that I became, at least for a brief while, Master Hu's unspoken, de facto, 'indoor student'.[2] Not long after this, with his encouragement, I began to offer Qigong classes for adults. In the past 25 years I have offered regular weekly classes for adults in many diverse locations (including a small pharmacy, a large university gym, a portable Nissan hut, various Yoga studios, a realtor's office, and outside by the lake) in various communities throughout Ontario, Canada.

By and large, most of the class participants have been relatively healthy and came to the classes to remain that way. Most were women aged 45–80, but occasionally my students, former students, participants' children, and the occasional man (usually a participant's partner or spouse) also participated.

Class size varied from 6–24 but on average 12 people were in class each week. Participants were very loyal attending for 3 or more years, and usually only stopped coming to class due to health problems (their own or family members), or relocation.

DOI: 10.4324/9780429439803-35

The class was designed to run for one hour with 50–55 minutes of exercise. I have run the class at various times throughout the day – e.g., at lunchtime (12.00–1.00), immediately after work (4.45–5.45, and early evening. However, for 12 years my class ran predominately in the early evening.

This worked especially well when conducted outside by the lake as we could watch the sun go down. In addition to my regular weekly classes, I ran weekend classes, Train The Trainer workshops, and programmes based on these weekly classes worldwide (including Australia, China, Portugal, New Zealand, South Africa, UK).

Programmes For People Living With Life-Threatening and Life-Changing Conditions[3]

> I am not this fragile body.[4]

In 1992, in addition to my academic movement classes, I started teaching Qigong and Tai Chi classes for the Campus Recreation programme at the University of Windsor. Through these classes I was introduced to the Windsor-Essex Cardiac Rehab Programme (WECRP), which operated in the same building, and was asked to teach a Qigong class. Participants were primarily recovering from a heart attack or stroke, but others were living with debilitating conditions such as lupus or rheumatoid arthritis.

Initially, I taught what I knew, a mixture of Tai Chi and standing Qigong forms learned from tapes and Western teachers I had encountered along the way. It didn't take me long to realise that the forms I was offering were wrong! I was teaching sets of exercises that did not make it easy for individuals to participate. The sets were too long, the exercises too strenuous, and, quite frankly, looking back I believe my sessions may have done more harm than good … but at the time I did not know how to fix it.

In 1993, as mentioned earlier, I became Master George Ling Hu's 'indoor student'. It was through Master Hu I first encountered seated Qigong. When first I experienced this, I thought it was interesting but didn't really see its relevance to either my teaching or personal practice. But my view of these exercises changed completely when I started to visit him in Houston. On these occasions I studied with Master Hu in his home and accompanied him to every session he ran. During these visits I had an epiphany.

Master Hu ran two classes that were for me somewhere between 'eye-opening' and 'jaw dropping'! The first was a session for cardiac rehab patients, which he taught in the weight room of a gym, by no means an ideal setting. The other was a seated Qigong class for seniors at a Methodist church in a very large auditorium of the kind one sees evangelical preachers use in their sermons on TV. Here I watched an extraordinary seated Qigong class with a group of seniors in which he got participants, many of whom were well over eighty, to move in ways that put my twenty-year-old university students to shame.

As I engaged in these exercises, some for the first time, I was intensely aware of not just what exercises he was using but also how he implemented them. His use of rhythm, the way he slowed the pace of the exercises to accommodate his elderly participants. The way he used pauses to enable participants to catch their breath and rest between and during exercises. The intense way he observed EVERYTHING without seeming to even be looking, to not give participants what he called 'eyeball pressure'. Most importantly the way he used humour and music. These teaching techniques, as much as the exercises themselves, had a profound effect on me.

Both these events changed me. They made me completely rethink the way I taught. As a result of this experience, I decided to teach seated Qigong classes. I began to lead Qigong classes for The Hospice of Windsor catering to persons with cancer and other life-threatening conditions. Later I began offering seated Qigong classes for The Windsor Essex Cardiac Rehab program. Over the years, participants in these two sets of classes have included people with Fibromyalgia, severe arthritis, MS, and victims of car accidents. Many participants had issues related to pain and cited Qigong as helping them with this.

Programmes For Seniors

In 2002 I started to run seated Qigong programmes for healthy seniors at the Jewish Community Centre in Windsor. Initially I ran these with my long-time assistant John Taylor. Later, I started to run similar programmes at the Windsor Centre for Seniors and at several seniors' residences. I ran these programmes for many years.

In 2011, I met with Mike Sharrat at a Sheridan College conference on ageing convened by Pat Spadafora. Mike and I discussed conducting research on the seated Qigong programme I had developed at various seniors' facilities and residences in Ontario.

As a result of these conversations in the summer of 2012 I began to offer seated Qigong programmes at a newly opened 'long-term care and retirement village' in Southwestern Ontario. This long-term care facility had just hired as their recreation coordinator a long-time colleague and supporter of my seated Qigong work with healthy seniors, and so it was an opportune moment to start this programme.

Research

The first research I did on seated Qigong was with participants on the Cardiac Rehab Qigong programme.[5] In the cardiac Qigong programme participants engaged in a 30–45-minute period of seated exercise with tranquil music playing in the background.[6] As with all courses offered by WECRP, blood pressure readings were taken before and after the class.

For our study, participants were also asked to answer a series of questions about their health during the previous week.[7] In addition, immediately before and after each class participants were asked to self-report in writing (using a simple seven-point-scale) about their level of pain, energy, relaxation, and how they felt overall. This information was monitored on a regular basis for both each individual and the class.

Our early research showed that thirty minutes of Qigong helps normalise blood pressure, lower pulse rate, and reduce stress as described by participant-administered assessment scale. We discovered significant positive short-term effects of seated Qigong participants' blood pressure and sense of wellbeing. This early research also showed that participants reported having more energy and less illness (shorter duration and less severe) and generally feeling healthier.[8]

In the first year of the research programme with seniors we conducted two different pieces of research – one for the pilot project, and one during the start-up phase of the seated Qigong programme. During both phases we collected qualitative observational data and quantitative data concerning pre- and post-blood pressures and heart rates.[9]

In time the programme became more established. The work, which began slowly with a 12-week pilot project continued through to my retirement from the University of Windsor in 2016. During this time, seated Qigong was delivered in three different neighborhoods[8] and in the library. The programme was very successful and led to the delivery of similar programmes at other long-term care facilities, several of which were led by Joanna Coughlin, who was instrumental in the development of the initial pilot programme.[10]

Notes

1 While specific exercises change from time to time, the programme follows a simple and similar pattern. This is the current sequence of exercise in my classes:

- Sinews Changing exercises
- Preparing The Body For Action
- Opening And Closing Breaths
- Ba Duan Jin
- Sinews Changing exercises – repeat
- Opening And Closing Breaths – repeat
- Cool Down.

2 Traditionally, martial arts masters took in 1–3 indoor students, who they taught one-to-one or in very small groups. These individuals, oftentimes their children, were taught the 'inside knowledge' – techniques and applications that were hidden from all other students. This included counters to attacks and the more devastating 'killing techniques' – e.g., Dim Mak, a secret body of knowledge with techniques

that attack pressure points and meridians, said to incapacitate or sometimes cause immediate or even delayed death to an opponent.

3 Much of what is written in this section appeared in a slightly different format in B. Warren (2017), Sit, Smile, Breathe: Seated Qigong for People with Life-changing Conditions: A Personal Reflection, *Journal of Complimentary Medicine and Alternative Healthcare* 1(3), https://juniperpublishers.com/jcmah/JCMAH.MS.ID.555562.php

4 Deng (1988).

5 While I occasionally added some 'wrinkles', the basic sequence for the Cardiac Rehab Qigong Programme was:

- Three Cleansing Breaths Qigong
- Balancing The Heart Qigong
- Triple Warmer Qigong
- Seated Bad Duan Jin
- Cool Down.

6 One feature of the programme was that the exercises were transportable, required no special equipment, and could be done by participants in their own time at home.

7 Participants were asked eight questions dealing with elements of physical health (e.g., heart rate, digestion) and emotional states (e.g., anxiety, depression, sense of wellbeing).

8 B. Warren and N. Gervais (2004), Sit, Breathe and Smile: The Short-term Effects of Qigong on Blood Pressure and Sense of Well-being for Cardiac Patients. Third Global Conference: Making Sense of Health, Illness and Disease. Oxford, England. July.

9 During the start-up phase Cheri McGowan and I carried out, and later published with others, significant research on the effects of the programme on blood pressure and quality of life. Freeman et al. (2014), https://pubmed.ncbi.nlm.nih.gov/24439645/

10 Further research and reflections on this work was published as B. Warren, J. Coughlin, M. Littlejohn, A. Campbell, and A. Warren (2018), https://juniperpublishers.com/jcmah/pdf/JCMAH.MS.ID.555673.pdf

Chapter 28

Exercises For Groups

This chapter builds on earlier chapters and is specifically for anyone who is leading movement workshops and classes with others. In it we describe six exercises specifically designed for groups.

Safety Tips For Group Movement

Freeze!

Freeze! should not be 'optional'. It is the instructor's greatest single safety tip, and participants need to learn it before any other work is undertaken. It is simple, effective, and truly the best crowd-control mechanism going.

- *Rule*: at any moment during the session, if the instructor calls *Freeze!*, participants must instantly stop and totally freeze. No questions, no excuses, no talking!
- Only when the instructor calls 'continue' do participants 'unfreeze' and continue with what they were doing.
- While considered an important safety 'device', *Freeze!* can also be used at any time during a class as an unexpected, fun element, to keep participants on their toes, or like a game, to enliven the mood.

Benefits:

- Since everyone participating is required to *Freeze!*, it effectively 'evens the playing field' between those with a lot of movement training and those with none or with serious disabilities.
- If people are working aggressively or in any way sabotaging the work, *Freeze!* allows instructors to avoid entanglements or negative contact and redirect with new exercises.
- It helps keep participants alert, focused, and in the moment.

DOI: 10.4324/9780429439803-36

Slow Motion ('Slo-Mo')

While excellent for 'exploring your body and space', slow motion can also be used as a safety device if a group is or is becoming too scattered, rowdy, confused, or aggressive as it instantly requires participants to concentrate deeply on what they are doing and how they are sculpting their movements in space.

- *Note*: the idea of slow motion also borrows liberally from Eastern-based movements.
- Slow motion does not mean that the group 'just slows down their movements'.
- All movements done in slow motion seem larger, more extended, almost 'inflated', and every part of the body seems more deliberate, directed, and internally driven – as if the whole body is involved in forwarding each action.
- To help achieve the 'feeling' and 'visuals' of slow motion, there are internal and external images that may help:

  a Full-body breathing will help and enhance slow motion actions
  b Think of the body trying to move while immersed in deep water
  c Internally, imagine the body is inflated, like a balloon and that every movement is internally pushed by air being forced into the moving parts.

Tip: remember to practise slow motion in lateral movements, backwards, turns, standing, and sitting!

Benefits:

- Can bring focus, clarity and control to the class when needed.
- It is surprisingly difficult and makes an excellent fitness training tool.
- Increases muscle and directional control.
- Exploring your body in space

  a Helps participants have time for practising connecting breathing to movement
  b Helps increase personal movement vocabulary
  c Increases spatial awareness of body and/in surroundings.

Centring and 'Shake-Outs'

- These movements are described in full in chapter 22, 'Reducing Stress'.
- They are excellent for preparing the body and the participants for group movement.
- They can be inserted at any time during the session to help participants focus, self-listen, relax, and breathe before continuing.

Benefits:

- *Centring* and *Shake-Outs* are always used together because Centring leaves people feeling truly 'anchored' to the spot and the Shake-Out redirects energy throughout the body, releases tension, and prepares the body for further movement activities.
- Instantly focuses participants to internal listening and 'seeing'.
- Slows down breathing and reduces blood pressure and muscular and emotional tension.

Group Activities

I Am Me

- Participants move around the room in a movement pattern of right foot stamp, left foot stamp, both feet jump.
- In each case, the hand (in the form of a clenched fist) cleaves through the air as the foot or feet contact the floor.
- The movement pattern is linked to a sequence of three words:

  a I (right foot stamp)
  b Am (left foot stamp)
  c Player's name (jump).

A variation is to remain seated, chanting the phrase, 'I, am, [players name]'.

Other Iteration Of This Game

This game can be played in two stages. In the first stage, the group stands in a large circle. In turn, each member of the group jumps in the air and as they land, they say their name – for example, 'Bernie'. The pace of this can slowly build until as soon as one person has landed the next person starts to jump, creating a 'jumping jack wall of sound'.

This leads on to the next stage, where the group moves as individuals around the room observing the following ritual. The ritual consists of a linked pattern of movements and words – for example, to make a personal statement about themselves:

Movement	*Stomp*	*Stomp*	*Jump*
Statements	I	Am	Susan
	I	Feel	happy
	I	want	ice cream

This sequence is repeated until you feel the group has had enough. The first part of the triad is always 'I am', but the second and third parts can be varied – for example, I need, I hate, I love, I fear ... according to the needs of your group.

In each case the statements are linked to the movement – for example:

Movement	*Stomp*	*Stomp*	*Jump*
Statements	I	Am	John
	I	Love	sleeping
	I	hate	work

In each case the statements are always individual and personal.

This game can be particularly valuable in enabling people to express their emotions vehemently without becoming 'spotlighted' or having the group focus on their problems, because their statements will be part of the group's 'wall of sound'.

Should you wish to bring the statements 'into the open', to be shared with the group, you can get the group back into a large circle and then ask each member of the group to cross the circle in the prescribed ritualised manner.

As leader you can choose which emotions you wish each person to describe, or this can be left up to members of the group. This can lead to group discussion or simply increase your store of information concerning the group.

Walk My Walk

This is empty space work that explores the ways the body can move.

Prison Yard Walks

Participants walk in a circle and are instructed to do one of the following (circle direction changes between types):

a Turn the feet out – walking faster
b Tight-rope walking – walking faster
c Turn feet in – walking faster
d Walk on outside edges of feet – walking faster
e Inside edges of feet – walking faster
f Placing magnet on parts of body – forehead, left shoulder, centre of breastbone, below belly button, dominant hip (pulse), non-dominant knee, big toe of dominant foot – rest of body resists.

Walk My Walk: Pair Work

This is done in stages:

a Observe and follow partner
b Place hand on the shoulder of partner and follow behind them
c Take the place of your partner – walking like your partner
d Find a new partner and try and absorb their learned walk
e Carry out guided action (the next activity) moving as their new character.

A Laban Story: Character Development/Working Story

As the character they have now taken on they will be guided through a story they are to act out.

- The story should hit the following points:

  a Climb stairs
  b Open door
  c Moving heavy box (push along floor)
  d Touch-up paint on a windowsill (using small light paintbrush)
  e Wring out clothing
  f Change quickly to meet beloved
  g Run downstairs and out the door
  h Struggle through tall grass and mud swatting mosquitoes as you go
  i Meet beloved
  j Ice skate
  k Fight vending machine for a drink of pop
  l Walk with beloved
  m Say goodbye
  n Go home.

- In twos, walk toward the mirror transitioning from character to back to self. When you reach the end say your name and something about yourself.

  Tip: can be very useful to discuss what it *felt like* to be in someone else's shoes.
  Benefits:

- Good transition into practical exploration of Laban's eight efforts
- Useful for teaching acting as it explores the concept that characters all have their own walks.

Precautions:

- Socks should be removed as they are a slipping hazard.

- It is important to give the participants the structured time to transition back into themselves.

Variation: instead of doing the walk of someone in the workshop/class, participants can go out and observe the walks of passers-by and copy those.

Vogue: Strike A Pose

- Gather the group together in a circle.
- Number participants off, alternately A and B.
- Call out an idea – e.g., war memorial
  - a All participants then run into the centre of the circle and strike a pose they think captures the idea
  - b Then return to their position in the circle.
- Continue calling out ideas but alternate between group A and group B entering the circle
  - a Each group is given a different idea but something similar or opposite) – e.g., famine, pleasure, pain, hockey, heroes, seaside/day at the beach, day at the spa, happiness, love.
- Continue for a few rotations.

Essence Machine: Moving Tableaux

Part 1:

Create groups of 4–5.
Ask each group to create an 8–12-second moving tableau that encapsulates an idea – e.g., breakfast, haunted house.
Ask each group to come up with topics for other groups.

Part 2:

Now look at the Taoist poems/meditations and haikus below.
Each group chooses one poem, then distils it into a silent moving tableau
Each group presents their interpretation of the poem *without* sharing what it is.

Part 3:

Groups now choose four or five words from their poems that they will speak while performing the moving tableau

a Can be same word or four different words
b Group can rechoreograph the movements to better fit with the words.

Each group may decide to

a Have one person say one word each
b Or speak words chorally
c Or a mixture of individual and choral for the 4–5 words.

Groups present their second distillation.
Groups then give feedback on this experience.

Benefits:

- Helps find the underlying meaning in large concepts.
- Explores and physicalises the emotion behind large-scale concepts.
- Finding the meaning in order to capitalise on it for scenes.
- The words can be changed depending on the mood or feeling of the lesson you are going for.

Precautions:

- Socks should be removed as they are slipping hazards.
- They may need more introduction into improvisation and physicalising large concepts if they have not had much introduction to movement and drama.
- Make sure that the poems used are not too long or it is too much to handle.

Taoist Poems

1	Make the crooked straight. Make the straight to flow. Gather water, fire, and light. Bring the world to a single point.	6	A solitary crane In winter snow Needs no jewels.
2	Arctic breath coils the mountain, Rattling the forests' bones. Raindrops cling to branches: Jewelled adornment flung to earth.	7	Lake shadows colour of cold, Willow branches weep ice, Swan rises dazzling in the sunlight.
3	Mute black night, Sudden fire. Destruction.	8	Wall of flames, bridge of tears. Snowflake on newly forged links.

4	Heron stands in the blue estuary, Solitary, white, unmoving for hours. A fish! Quick avian darting; The prey captured.	9	Enter the cavern with its Walls of tangled strands. Find the living flame. That burns on blood.
5	Storm breaks into pieces, Clouds charge the horizon. Revolving of the heavens Generates all movement.	10	Powdered concubine dressed in rich silks – Feet bound, body, soft, lips slack – Views lotuses through binoculars. A dragonfly alights on her motionless fan.

(From Ming-Dao Deng, 1988)

Increasing Movement Vocabulary

One of the best ways to keep our bodies agile and responsive is through exploring and expanding our *movement vocabulary.* This involves pushing the boundaries of our daily set movement patterns by adding some fun, imagination, and the unexpected to the mix. There are literally endless examples that we can use – people, nature, cooking actions, to name just a few.
Here are two variations: *Copycat Circles* and *Movement Mix-Ups.*

Copycat Circles

This is a fun, easily adapted, and effective way of expanding our 'regular' patterns of moving and observing, as well as improving reflexes. It can have many variations.

- As the title suggests, have the group stand in a large circle.
- Give group a 'prompt' to use, such as popcorn popping, balloon exploding, smoke rising, one slow motion fake karate move, slo-mo happy cheer, waves in a storm, fake chorus line dance move, etc., etc.
- One single prompt continues to be used as the source for each person in the circle's 'movement offer'.
- Play with slow and fast tempos and include different directions, but the prompts should always suggest *large* movements.
- Indicate who will begin 'offering' one large, imaginative movement, and in which direction the next 'offer' will come (clockwise or counter clockwise).
- To ensure that people are not holding their breath and that their breathing is as large as and in keeping with the physical movement, have the

offer-mover make a large *sound* (note: not an actual word – just a sound!) that accompanies the offered movement.

- On a signal from the instructor, the first pre-decided person performs an 'offer' sound-and-movement, which is large, clear, and done once only.
- Note: at the end of each offer, the offer-performer *freezes* in position.
- The *moment* the offer-performer is 'frozen,' all other participants repeat the offer sound-and-movement *simultaneously*, including the 'freeze' ending in their response.
- Note: their *response should happen immediately*, so they are working to improve their response/reflex timing and learning to override their 'critical editor'.
- Response-participants *reproduce* the offer sound-and-movement as closely as possible.
- At the exact moment that the responders freeze, the next 'offer-mover' gives a new example. The immediacy of this new offer is important in order not to 'overthink' and to 'override' perfectionist tendencies about 'doing it right'.

Precautions:

- Make sure there is sufficient room between participants so that they can do large movements.
- Always remind people to adjust to their capacities and to not 'overdo' a movement that might re-injure or overly stress them in any way.
- If any participant seems eager to invade others' space, be prepared to call "Freeze!"[1]
- If the space is very limited, divide participants into two groups, having one group work while the others actively watch.

Tips:

- 'Active' watching[2] can be very helpful and informative for participants. Even if there is room for everyone to work simultaneously, once the group is comfortable with each other, you may choose to divide group into 'watchers' and 'movers'.
- If you divide the group, switch up each time a circle of 'offers' has been completed.

Benefits: this exercise works at many levels, giving participants more practice at

- Connecting breathing and movement to imagination and fun
- Increasing personal movement (and sound) vocabulary
- Increasing reflexes

- Gaining confidence and lessening their 'mind critics' hold on 'right and wrong'.

Movement Mix-Ups[3]

This is a whimsical, unexpected, and fun exercise that can be done with small to very large groups. Again, each movement response is open to personal interpretation – there is no right or wrong answer.

Step 1: One body part + one verb

- These lists can be written on the board or on paper or be put on separate ballots in different hats or jars … or 'made up' on the spot.
- The instructor randomly chooses a) one body part and b) one verb (no 'pre-determining' pairings! This is about celebrating the unexpected).
- Participants are to move randomly around the room, combining the body part and the verb. Note: yes, whimsical, weird, fun, unexpected … .
- Change up pairings quickly – never give participants time to get bored.

List of Body Parts

Hands and wrists	Arms	Hands and tummies
Fingers	Tummy and back	Tummy and back
Feet and ankles	Elbows and hands	Shoulders
Shoulders	Elbows and knees	Hips (do separately)
Knees	Back of head	Whole body
Head	Legs and feet	

Verbs (body, nature, other)

Giggle	Scream	Burp
Smirk	Roar	Swallow
Cough	Sneeze	Soar
Yawn	Swallow	Crinkle
Hiccup	Chew	Fold
Flap		

Step 2: One body part + one verb + add directional instructions

Once participants are familiar with the exercise, add directions to be done simultaneously. Here are just some possibilities:

- ... while moving in semi-circles
- ... while moving in slow or fast zigzags
- ... while moving in wavy lines forward, backwards, side to side, in circles
- ... while moving in squares
- ... while moving in triangles.

Tips:

- Remember, there is no right or wrong!
- Before starting exercise and after 'Freeze!', be sure to do a fast *Shake-Out*.

Precautions:

- Keep a distance from walls, furniture, and other participants – this is a no-contact sport!
- Always obey instantly if/when the instructor calls 'Freeze!'

Step 3: Images invoking movement quality

Once participants are familiar with the exercise, you can add images that invoke a quality of movement to be interpreted by participants. Here are a few possibilities:

Steam rising	*Lightning*	*Wind whistling*
Wet spaghetti	Thunder clouds	Raging waves
Popcorn	Beating rain	Butterfly flying
Bubbling porridge	Campfire	Cat stretching
Candle	Mist rolling	

Benefits:

- This multi-layered exercise increases
  - a Spatial and body awareness
  - b Movement vocabulary and reflex responses
  - c Confidence in moving
  - d Ability to override and ignore our 'critical' perfectionist inner voice.

Notes

1 'Freeze!' is the group instructor's best friend: always make groups aware that at *any* moment that the instructor calls 'Freeze!', all participants must stop instantly – like frozen statues.

2 *Active* watching, as it suggests, means watching participants are to carefully observe their peers moving in order to be aware of what is expected and better prepared once they return to 'moving' from 'watching'.
3 An exercise invented by Jean-Pierre Gauthier, Lecoq peer and founding member of Theatre Action, Auckland, NZ.

References and Further Reading

Axline, V. (1947). *Play Therapy.* New York: Ballantine Books.

Bartenieff, I. (1980). *Body Movement: Coping with the Environment.* New York: Gordon & Breach.

Barton, J. and Pretty, J. (2010). What is the Best Dose of Nature and Green Exercise for Improving Mental Health? A Multi-Study Analysis. *Environmental Science & Technology* 44(10): 3947–3955.

Beckett , S. (1956). *Waiting for Godot.* London: Faber & Faber.

Berger, J. (1972). *Ways of Seeing.* London: Penguin.

Blatner, A. (1997). *Acting-In: Practical Applications of Psychodramatic Methods.* London: Free Association.

Breitenbecher, K.H., and Fuegen, K. (2019). Nature and Exercise Interact to Influence Perceived Restorativeness. *Ecopsychology* 11(1): 34–42.

Brook, P. (1968). *The Empty Space.* London: Penguin.

Brown, S. (2009). *Play: How it Shapes the Brain, Opens the Imagination and Invigorates the Soul.* New York: Avery.

Capra, F. (1975). *The Tao of Physics: An Exploration of the Parallels between Modern Physics and Eastern Mysticism.* London: Wildwood House.

Callois, R. (2001). *Man, Play and Games.* Reprint edn. Champaign: University of Illinois Press.

Cohen, D. (1987). *The Development of Play.* Beckenham, Kent: Croom Helm.

Deng, M.-D. (1988). *365 Tao: Daily Meditations.* New York: Harper.

Egoscue, P., and Gittines, R. (2000). *Pain Free: A Revolutionary Method for Stopping Chronic Pain.* New York: Random House.

Exley, H. (ed.) (1981). *What It's Like to Be Me.* Watford: Exley Publications.

Feldenkrais, M. (1972). *Awareness Through Movement.* New York: Harper Collins.

Field, S.L. (2003). *The Zangshu, or Book of Burial.* Transl. In *Fengshui Gate.* http://faculty.trinity.edu/sfield/Fengshui/Zangshu.html.

Frantzis, B (2005). *Opening the Energy Gates of Your Body: Qigong for Lifelong Health.* Berkeley, CA: Blue Snake Books.

Frantzis, B. (2012). *Bagua and Tai Chi: Exploring the Potential of Chi, Martial Arts, Meditation, and the I Ching.* Berkeley: Blue Snake Books.

Gardner, H. (1983). *Frames of Mind: A Theory of Multiple Intelligences.* New York: Basic Books.

Gascon, M., Zijlema, W., Vert, C., White, M.P., and Nieuwenhuijsen, M.J. (2017). Outdoor Blue Spaces, Human Health and Well-being: A Systematic Review of Quantitative Studies. *International Journal of Hygiene and Environmental Health* 220(8): 1207–1221.

Glasbergen, R. (2006). *Weird and Wonderful World of Work*. Lagoon Books.

Gordon, D. (1978). *Therapeutic Metaphors: Helping Others Through the Looking Glass*. Chicago: Meta Publications.

Hanna, J.L. (2006). *Dancing for Health: Conquering and Preventing Stress*. Lanham, MD: AltaMira Press.

Hoff, B. (1982). *The Tao of Pooh*. London: Penguin.

Huzinga, J. (1955). *Homo Ludens: A Study of the Play Element in Culture*. Boston, MA: Beacon Press.

Jahnke, R., Larkey, L., Rogers, C., Etnier, J., and Fang, L. (2010). A Comprehensive Review of Health Benefits of Qigong and Tai Chi. *American Journal of Health Promotion* 24(6): e1–e25.

Kahane, A., and Barnum, J. (2017). *Collaborating with the Enemy: How to Work with People You Don't Agree With or Like or Trust*. www.books24x7.com/marc.asp?bookid=120323.

Kisselgoff, A. (1957). Ballet: Graham's 'Persephone'. *New York Times*, 15 October 1987, Section C, Page 23. www.nytimes.com/1987/10/15/arts/ballet-graham-s-persephone.html.

Klate, J. (1980). *The TAO of Acupuncture*. Ann Arbor, MI: UMI.

Korzybski, A. (1995). *Science and Sanity: An Introduction to Non-Aristotelian Systems and General Semantics*. 5th edn. New York: Institute of General Semantics.

Laban, R. (1971). *The Mastery of Movement*. London: Macdonald & Evans.

Lecoq, J. (2006). *Theatre of Movement and Gesture*. Oxon: Routledge.

Lerman, L. (1980). *Teaching Dance to Senior Adults*. Springfield, IL: C. Thomas.

Levete, G. (1982). *No Handicap to Dance*. London: Souvenir Press.

Little, S., and Eichman, S. (2000). *Taoism and the Arts of China*. Chicago: Art Institute of Chicago; Berkeley/Los Angeles: University of California Press.

Master Lam (1991). *The Way of Energy: Mastering the Chinese Art of Internal Strength with Chi Kung Exercise*. New York: Simon & Schuster.

Mate, G. (1999). *Scattered Minds: A New Look at the Origins and Healing of Attention Deficit Disorder*. Ist edn. Toronto: Knopf Canada.

Mate, G. (2011). *When the Body Says No: Understanding the Stress-Disease Connection*. Hoboken, NJ: Wiley.

McLuhan, M. (1964). *Understanding Media: The Extensions of Man*. New York: McGraw-Hill.

MoraMarco, J., and Benzel, R. (2000). *The Way of Walking*. Chicago: Contemporary Books.

North, M. (1972). *Personality Assessment through Movement*. London: Macdonald & Evans.

Powers, S. (2008). *Insight Yoga: An Innovative Synthesis of Traditional Yoga, Meditation, and Eastern Approaches to Healing and Well-Being*. Boulder, CO: Shambhala Publications.

Preston-Dunlop, V. (1988). *Handbook for Dance in Education*. Saddle River, NJ: Pearson Education.

Qing Li (2018). *Forest Bathing: How Trees Can Help You Find Health and Happiness.* New York: Viking.

Sagli, G. (2008). Learning and Experiencing Chinese Qigong in Norway. *East Asian Science* 2: 545–566.

Slade, P. (1977). *Natural Dance.* London: Hodder Arnold.

Stein, P. (2004). Representation, Rights, and Resources: Multimodal Pedagogies in the Language and Literacy Classroom. In *Critical Pedagogies and Language Learning*, edited by B. Norton and K. Toohey. New York: Cambridge University Press.

Sutton-Smith, B. (1979). *Play and Learning.* New York: Gardner Press.

Thompson Coon, J., Boddy, K., Stein, K., Whear, R., Barton, J., and Depledge, M.H. (2011). Does Participating in Physical Activity in Outdoor Natural Environments Have a Greater Effect on Physical and Mental Wellbeing than Physical Activity Indoors? A Systematic Review. *Environmental Science & Technology* 45(5): 1761–1772.

Robbie, S., and Warren, B. (2020). Dramatising the Shock of the New: Using Arts-based Embodied Pedagogies to Teach Life Skills. *Discourse: Studies in the Cultural Politics of Education*, doi:10.1080/01596306.2020.1843114.

Seale, A. (2016). The Liminal Space: Embracing the Mystery and Power of Transition from What Has Been to What Will Be. *Center for Transformational Presence*, 24 October. https://transformationalpresence.org/alan-seale-blog/liminal-space-embracing-mystery-power-transition-will-2/.

Shakespeare, W. (1603). *The Tragicall History of Hamlet Prince of Denmarke.* First Quarto. Reprint Clarendon Press, 1957. Most modern texts and performances are based on the Second Quarto of 1604/5.

Sheng, Ken Yun (1997). *Walking Kung.* Newburyport, MA: Samuel Weiser.

Sweeney, E. (ed.) (2023). *Space, Place and Dramatherapy.* London: Routledge.

Veith, I. (2002). *Huang Ti Nei Ching Su Wên: The Yellow Emperor's Classic of Internal Medicine.* Oakland, CA: University of California Press.

Warren, B. et al. (2018). Seeking The Dragon's Pearl: Reflections on the Benefits of Tai-jiquan and Qigong for University Students. *International Journal of Complementary and Alternative Medicine* 11(2): 57–60. https://medcraveonline.com/IJCAM/seeking-the-dragons-pearl-reflections-on-the-benefits-of-taijiquan–qigong-for-university-students.html.

Warren, B. (1988). *Disability And Social Performance. Using Drama To Achieve Successful 'Acts Of Being'.* Cambridge, MA: Brookline Books.

Warren, B. (1997). Change and Necessity: Creative Activity, Well-being, and the Quality of Life for Persons with a Disability. In *Quality Of Life For People With A Disability*, edited by R.I. Brown, 270–291. Cheltenham: Stanley Thornes.

Warren, B. (ed.) (2008). *Using The Creative Arts in Therapy and Healthcare.* 3rd ed. Oxon: Routledge.

Warren, B. (2011). *Drama Games (revisited): A Practical Introduction to Drama Games and Activities for People of All Ages and Abilities.* Concord, ON: Captus Press.

Warren, B. (2022). *Teddy Teaches Tai Chi.* Illust. by A Simioni. Cavan, ON: YGT-Media Co.

Warren, B., and Coaten, R. (2008). Dance: Developing Self-image and Self-expression Through Movement. In *Using the Creative Arts in Therapy and Healthcare*, edited by B. Warren, 64–88. Oxon: Routledge.

Warren, B., and Coughlin, J. (2014). *Stand, Breathe, Smile: Simple Standing Exercises and Approaches to Reduce Stress and Promote Good Health*. Marietta, GA: Tranquility Press.

Warren, B., and Spitzer, P. (2014). *Smiles Are Everywhere: Integrating Clown-Play into Healthcare Practice*. London and New York: Routledge.

Warren, B., Robbie, S., Gilbert, K.E., and Taylor, J.(2019). Lovely by the Water: Reflections on the Pleasures and Benefits of Doing Qigong in Natural Surroundings. *Journal of Complementary & Alternative Medicine* 10(3): 555787. www.researchgate.net/publication/335841419_Lovely_by_the_Water-_Reflections_on_the_Pleasures_and_Benefits_of_Doing_Qigong_in_Natural_Surroundings.

Way, B. (1967). *Development Through Drama*. London: Longmans.

Weiger, L., and Bryce, D. (eds/transls) (1984). *Wisdom of the Daoist Masters: The Works of Lao Zi (Lao Tzu), Lie Zi (Lieh Tzu), Zhuang Zi (Chuang Tzu)*. Burnham-on-Sea, UK: Llanerch Press.

Winnicott, D.W. (1971). *Playing and Reality*. London: Tavistock.

Index

Note: Locators followed by "n" indicate endnotes.

For Product Safety Concerns and Information please contact our EU representative GPSR@taylorandfrancis.com
Taylor & Francis Verlag GmbH, Kaufingerstraße 24, 80331 München, Germany

www.ingramcontent.com/pod-product-compliance
Ingram Content Group UK Ltd.
Pitfield, Milton Keynes, MK11 3LW, UK
UKHW020139200926
475702UK00005B/815
* 9 7 8 1 1 3 8 3 4 2 2 8 6 *